TRAIL BLAZING

PRAISE FOR *TRAILBLAZING*

"Over a lifetime of running, I've pretty much seen it all.

The highs of Olympic and World Championship glory; the lows of devastating injury, disappointment, and failure; forging lifelong friendships and bonds just through running together; and the loneliness of having to struggle by yourself; and especially the pride and self-worth that comes from achieving the simple but difficult.

All these insights and emotions are covered in this humanistic, scientific, inspiring, and honest read.

Congratulations, Jenson, for sharing your story, because running is not a sport; it's a lifestyle, and the marathon a journey of liberation and self-discovery that we all should go on.

I know this book will inspire many to have the courage to try."

ROBERT DE CASTELLA
AO MBE, Australian former world champion
marathon runner and Olympian

"Having shared the trails with Jenson during UTA100 in 2022, I was immediately struck by his passion, enthusiasm and the important part that running plays in his life story. This is the amazing thing that draws you into the running community: the inspirational people you meet and the experiences you get to share and work through during the dizzying highs and terrifying lows. Congratulations Jenson on this amazing achievement and sharing your journey."

NICK PING
Outdoor and ultra-trail running enthusiast

"Jenson's infectious charisma and encouraging personality are like a second wind to any burgeoning runner. His personal journey to health through running is nothing short of inspirational."

BEN JAMES
Science teacher, St. Edmund's College

TRAIL BLAZING

HOW TO TAKE CONTROL OF YOUR HEALTH, VITALITY AND LONGEVITY THROUGH RUNNING

JENSON "THE RUN DOC" MAK
MBBS PhD FRACP FARM FACP

First published in 2023 by Dean Publishing
PO Box 119
Mt. Macedon, Victoria, 3441
Australia
deanpublishing.com

DEAN PUBLISHING

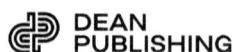

Cataloguing-in-Publication Data
National Library of Australia
Title: Trailblazing: How to take control of your health, vitality and longevity through running
Edition: 1st edn
ISBN: 978-1-925452-72-3
Category: Health and Fitness/Running/Longevity

DEDICATION

As I complete my maiden book, *Trailblazing*, I'm about to embark on one of the biggest challenges in my running career – and in my life – thus far. I'm talking about the 171-kilometre (106-mile) Ultra Trail du Mont-Blanc (UTMB) on 1–2 September 2023, where I'll be starting a mammoth route from Chamonix, France, and will traverse into Italy and Switzerland before making the counterclockwise loop back to Chamonix. The UTMB is regarded as one of the most challenging trail running events in the world. Essentially, it's the holy grail of trail ultramarathons.

I would like to dedicate this book to my late grandmother, FC Wong, who taught me the importance of strategising and adopting a positive mindset for problem-solving.

I also dedicate this book to my late mother, Demi, who instilled in me the 'KIA KAHA' warrior spirit and stressed the importance of people skills and effective communication.

I know that both my mother and grandmother will be the sun and the moon guiding me through the 10,000-metre mountain peak adventure I'll soon be tackling.

Finally, I pay my respect to the Elders past and present and extend that respect to all Aboriginal and Torres Strait Islander peoples today, especially to the Guringai people on Garigal land on which I've trained for most of my trail runs.

TABLE OF CONTENTS

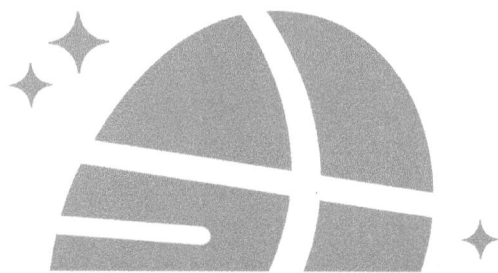

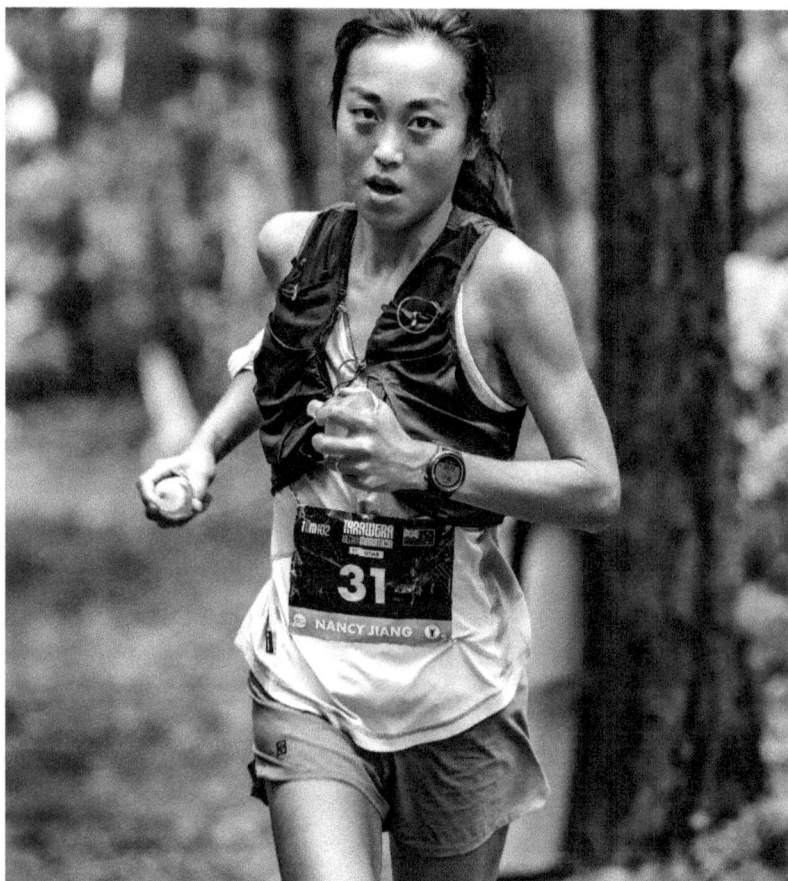

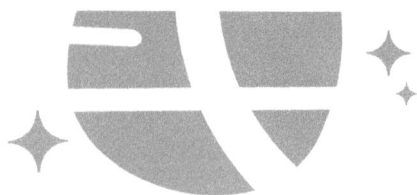

Nancy Jiang

FOREWORD

NANCY JIANG

Nancy Jiang is a structural engineer who was born in China and migrated to New Zealand at 5 years old. She represented New Zealand at the World Mountain Running Championships and the World Trail Running Championships and was the first female finisher at the 2023 Tarawera Ultramarathon 102 km.

I grew up in a traditional Chinese household, where everyone wished each other good health and good wealth. Striving for good wealth was well taken care of, with emphasis on studying, getting the best grades possible, aiming for top of the class and no less. But what about health? That also doesn't magically appear on its own. I'm forever grateful to my strong-minded self that I chose to also look after my health. And I'm not just talking about BMI (body mass index) or cholesterol ratio sort of health; I'm talking about mental health and happiness of the mind.

When I chose to run at school, it was purely because I enjoyed it and got a kick out of being faster than my peers.

Since then, being healthy and taking time to be outdoors in nature has always been an integral part of my life. Running has taken me on quite a life journey – from running barefoot across the sports field at a primary school cross-country competition to running up a 3000-metre-high mountain in Andorra, wearing the New Zealand (NZ) silver fern singlet, to participating in the world's oldest 100-mile foot race, the Western States Endurance Run.

We all know that exercise is good for our health, and running is one of the simplest ways to add more movement to our lives. It doesn't matter if you can only manage a 1-kilometre walk around the block to begin with because I can guarantee you that what you're able to do now certainly won't be what you'll be able to do in a year's time, a month, or even a week. The first step is often the hardest. I hope Jenson's story will give you the motivation to take ownership of your health and embark on your own running journey. Who knows where this journey will take you?

"Running well is a matter of having the patience to persevere when we are tired and not expecting instant results."

– Robert 'Deek' de Castella

INTRODUCTION

OUR RUN BEGINS

Before the dawn of the running revolution, our prehistoric ancestors, Homo sapiens sapiens, were already proficient at running. They ran long distances, barefoot, through the savannas of Africa to hunt for their next meal. They sprinted towards their prey to catch it and take it down. Finally, they carried the carcass all the way back to the safety of their cave to share with the tribe.

Meanwhile, in 2015, a 39-year-old, overweight, sedentary, middle-aged Asian man from Hong Kong, who couldn't even walk up a flight of stairs without panting, was experiencing an existential moment. After deciding that enough was enough, he was about to take a crucial step towards changing his own destiny and altering the lives of the people around him.

Introducing the Run Doc…

Hey, I'm Jenson Mak, also known as the Run Doc, and I'm here to show you a novel yet simple way to the holy grail of longevity. I'm a medical specialist, clinician, and researcher, but I'm also an ultramarathon runner and running coach. As of writing, I've run 40 marathons, 6 ultramarathons, including a 100-kilometre race, and helped over 10,000 patients in my clinical practice over the span of 23 years.

As Tony Robbins once said, "If you can recognize PATTERNS, you have an edge. No matter the situation – you'll recognize the pattern, learn how to use it, create something new, and DOMINATE."[1] At my weakest and darkest hour of subhealth (suboptimal health), as I stared lovingly into the eyes of my helpless newborn child, I felt a sudden desperation to cling to my life for an extra second, minute, hour, day, week, month, decade so I could spend quality time with my family and friends, enjoy the fruits of my labour, and explore the natural wonders of the world.

Also, I recognised a pattern. What was this pattern? Those who were physically active, going back as far as our ancient ancestors, were also healthy. I didn't need a pill or a procedure to solve my problem because the world's best medicine was, in fact, programmed into our DNA. I had already seen my first two children grow up, run free, and be happy and healthy. The concept isn't new, but it's something many of us have forgotten. *Why shouldn't I harness the primal power of physical activity to better my own health and happiness?*

To me, the solution was clear. *Running.* Running was the answer.

Since then, the Run Doc running philosophy has improved the lives of thousands of clients, including me – guinea pig number one.

In an age when social media and pushers of fad diets imply that fit, well-sculpted bodies can be chiselled overnight, we need to cut through the nonsense and get real about our health and fitness. Without the correct training and advice, a runner's physique (both physically and mentally) is impossible to achieve. It may be tough to hear, but there are no shortcuts. If you want to be fit and healthy, you must be prepared to do the work. Fortunately, you've shown serious initiative simply by picking up this book, so I'm here to guide you from wherever you are now on your running journey all the way to the finish line.

In *Trailblazing: How to Take Control of Your Health, Vitality and Longevity through Running*, among many other insights, I share the four pillars of the Run Doc running philosophy:

1. Unlock your healthy ageing and take the path to longevity, no matter where you are on the health spectrum.

2. Unleash your best self so you can become a healthier, happier, and more holistic version of your current self.

3. Align your mind-body-heart connection through running so you can run with ease, regardless of your fitness level.

4. Unwind the ageing clock and gain years on your life through cardio fitness.

Trailblazing's 11 chapters (the number representing my 'uniquely shaped' running legs) will take you on a journey of discovery as you become intimately familiar with the Run Doc philosophy. At the end of each chapter, I'll also provide a list of Run Doc tips to summarise my thoughts and reflections.

I wrote this book to share my personal journey, to show how I went from the Fat Doc to the Run Doc, and to teach the concept of healthy ageing. I also aim to make my clients and fellow clinicians aware of the inherent dangers of latent coronary artery disease and stroke and to prevent its occurrence through running and other aerobic activities.

Are you ready to be your best self? Let's get running together!

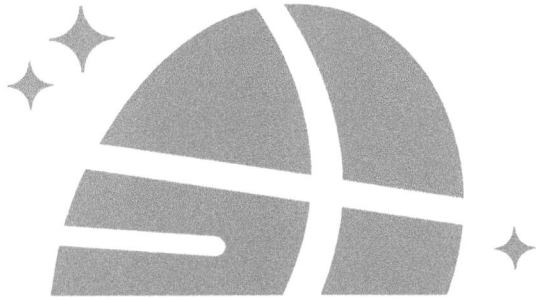

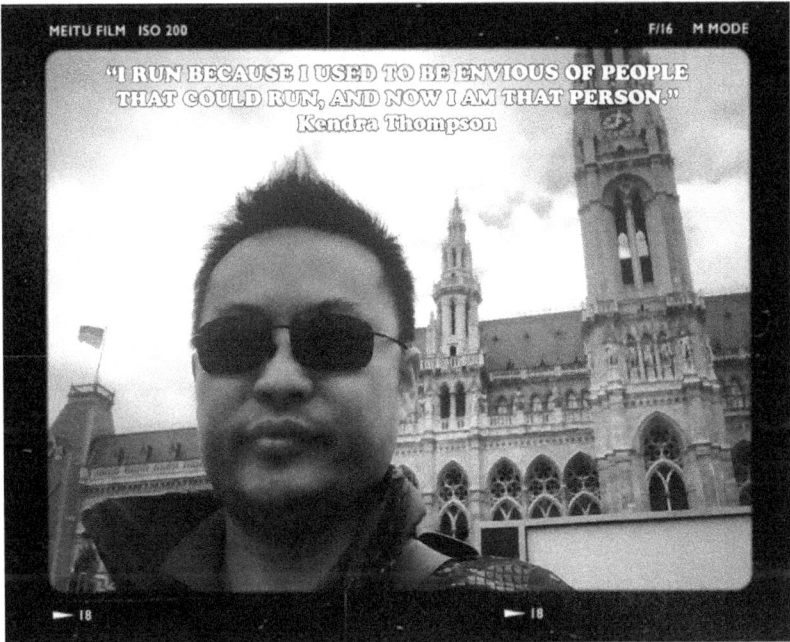

MEITU FILM   ISO 200 F/16   M MODE

"I RUN BECAUSE I USED TO BE ENVIOUS OF PEOPLE
THAT COULD RUN, AND NOW I AM THAT PERSON."
Kendra Thompson

18 18

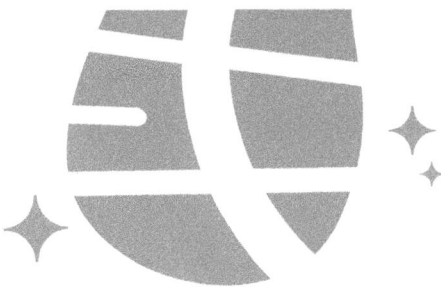

"I am not quite the fastest runner of the bunch, but I can run far, and that's my superpower!"

– The Run Doc

CHAPTER 1

====

GET HOOKED ON THE WORLD'S MOST POWERFUL PILL

At the ripe old age of 39, I was seemingly at the top of my game. My third child had miraculously arrived on Earth, and I was secure in my profession as an established medical specialist, with a good income to support my family. But I wasn't happy.

Beneath the joyful exterior of fun-loving, successful doctor lay 'the Fat Doc': overweight, hypertensive, chronically sleep-deprived, overworked, suffering from fatty liver disease, obstructive sleep apnoea, chronic stress, anxiety, and borderline depression. With such a laundry list of health problems, it's a wonder I was able to maintain a smile at all. Clearly, something had to change.

Now You Know My Secret... I Used to be The Fat Doc

My transition from fit to fat took place over many years and was so gradual and subtle I didn't even notice it was happening. Three key events, three *realisations*, caused me to make a radical life change and go from the Fat Doc to the Run Doc, a much more flattering title – wouldn't you agree?

1. I realised I was the Fat Doc

When I was at my fattest, I was getting a lot of headaches, among other telltale signs that something was wrong. I didn't want to admit it at the time, but I was overweight, unfit, and in bad health. However, I soon received a big dose of reality when I kept failing a blood pressure test for an insurance policy renewal. At that point, I was a successful, practising doctor, and I wasn't used to failing tests, especially one as important as a *blood pressure test*, so I was a little shocked at the results. I mean, I was fat, but I wasn't *that* fat, was I? Regardless, my blood pressure rating was through the roof, so whatever I was wasn't great for my health and wellbeing.

Years of minimal aerobic exercise, a penchant for devouring anything sweet, especially chocolate (often for stress relief or boredom), and a poor sleep pattern (from heavy on-call commitments) had taken a toll on my mind and body. Physically, I was overweight, almost 20 kg heavier than my fittest – that's two gigantic bags of 10 kg rice strapped on my body 24 hours a day! Mentally, I was in a chronically stressed state, constantly feeling fatigued and lacklustre.

I was a doctor; people's health was in my hands, but I wasn't taking responsibility for my own health. To me, that seemed hypocritical. Who was going to trust a fat doc who got short of breath walking from the car to the office, and who couldn't walk up a flight of stairs without getting palpitations? I wasn't exactly the best person to be giving health advice, especially when the results of multiple failed blood pressure tests showed that my own health was less than optimal.

2. I realised I couldn't keep up with my 7-year-old daughter

To further prove my poor health and fitness, my 7-year-old daughter asked me to help train her for her annual school cross-country race. Technically, I was a runner in high school and ran four consecutive City2Surfs (an annual 14-km road race from Sydney's CBD to the iconic Bondi Beach), so I thought I would make a good coach.

We went to Bert Oldfield Oval, a local dog park, and started jogging. I tried to keep up with her, but I couldn't. I was puffed out after 300 metres, and I had to stop. To save face, I pretended I had stopped so I could coach her better, and I quickly headed back to the starting line, which was also our agreed finishing point. I was thoroughly embarrassed at how out of shape I had gotten, and I didn't want my daughter to realise I couldn't keep up with her.

She later qualified to represent her zone in the cross-country championships and was eventually chosen to represent her entire school as the cross-country captain, one of her achievements I'm most proud of.

3. I realised I wanted to be there for my family

When my youngest son was born, I really started to notice the poor physical state I had gotten myself into – as if I didn't already know! After the birth, he was resting on my belly, looking up at me, so small, so helpless. We connected. Suddenly, I saw a flash of the future, and I realised I wanted to see him grow up. I wanted to see him graduate, get married, maybe have a kid of his own one day as I become a grand-parent. I wanted to be there for him through every milestone of his life. I wanted to be there for my other children too, and for my partner.

Clearly, I couldn't continue along the path I was on if I wanted to be the fit, healthy father my kids needed. I had a big problem, and, although I didn't realise it immediately, running was the solution. When I finally admitted I was maybe, perhaps, quite possibly a bit on the chunky side, I was 39 years old. I was coming to the end of another decade, pushing 40. It's a time in many people's lives when they decide to start running marathons. As it turned out, I was no different.

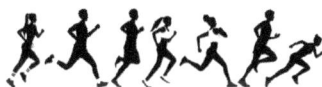

An Unlikely Place to Resume Running

When I started running again, I did so in an unlikely place: on a cruise ship. I was cruising the Pacific Island with my parents, and I was bored. Most of the time, we were waiting to get to an island, and I had nothing to do — Zumba and linedancing weren't my passions! I noticed people running laps on the top deck, and I felt compelled to join them, so I started jogging. At the time, I had zero motivation to run, so I popped on some headphones, selected a playlist of my favourite songs, and tried to disassociate from the unpleasant experience of physically exerting myself.

As I ran, I had flashbacks to my earlier years, finishing at the back of the pack in cross-country training and struggling my way through the City2Surf, but still finishing with an okay time. However, after the first lap of the deck, which was probably around 200 metres, I felt pretty good, and I pushed myself to do five laps in total to make my run exactly 1 kilometre long.

The next day, I told myself I would feel *really* good if I did ten laps – and I was right. I did feel good. The bonus was that I had an audience: bikini-clad young ladies, mums and dads, fit gym junkies, tanned and fit grandparents, and everyone else, all giving me high fives and verbal encouragement. Every "good job, mate" made the experience more enjoyable and spurred me to continue. Mentally, each lap I completed triggered my inner reward system. Running felt *great*.

By the end of the five-day cruise, I had fallen in love with running and the positive feelings that came with it. When I got home, I continued to train at the local dog park, which was a fairly flat area – perfect! During each run, I felt like I was dying, but, to my surprise, I always survived. Afterwards, I was huffing, puffing, and thankful it was over. However, within the next hour, I noticed something strange. I felt amazing. I soon realised that the longer I ran, the more euphoric I felt afterwards. After running 1 kilometre, I felt great, so I started to wonder what 5 kilometres would feel like. What would 10 kilometres feel like? What about a marathon? The euphoria I felt after running kept me coming back for more, and I gradually increased the distance I ran.

I also received some motivation from the Runkeeper running app, with the dulcet tones of Drill Instructor or Mademoiselle gently persuading, keeping me on track, telling how many kilometres I had run. Watching my 7-min/km pace go down to 6 minutes 45 seconds and lower gave me an external motivator to continue pushing for improvement.

Was I addicted? Maybe. But it was a positive addiction – much better than chowing down on chocolate or guzzling wine – and I was experiencing a clear physical transformation.

From a 5-km run, I progressed to completing my first 10-km event and signed up for my first half marathon, the Sydney Morning Herald (now HOKA) Half Marathon, raising over $12,000 for neurological research at NeuRA. I ended up being one of the top fundraisers, which gave me even more incentive to train and complete the race.

Over a three-month period, the weight fell off – 20 kg of fat as well as countless inches of middle-age spread. During this time, I also changed my eating habits, which were a big contributor to my weight gain. As my body grew healthier, so did my mind, and I was better able to manage my over-enjoyment of food, which had previously included plenty of chocolate and alcohol. Really, I replaced several unhealthy habits with one healthful addiction, and I saw the benefits almost immediately. Finally, I was on the path from the Fat Doc to the Fit – no, I was the *Run Doc*. But my journey was just beginning.

The Magic Pill (Benefits of Aerobic Exercise)

Out of all the medications and interventions I've ever prescribed, undeniably, aerobic exercise is the most powerful.

To date, over 500,000 scholarly articles have been published on 'aerobic exercise', including almost 70,000 clinical trials, with over 50,000 being randomised controlled trials, which are of the highest academic calibre. Meta-analyses consistently find that aerobic exercise benefits every single organ and system in the body, from the endocrine system to the brain.

In one meta-analysis, researchers found that regular aerobic exercise reduced waist circumference and visceral body fat and that higher-intensity training achieved the best results.[2] So, if you're looking to shed some weight, specifically body fat, aerobic exercise is the ideal complement to a good diet.

Okay, so that's an example of the physical benefits. But what about the mental benefits? I don't call aerobic exercise a magic pill for nothing. In another study, researchers concluded that aerobic exercise promotes positive mental and physical changes in people with schizophrenia.[3] On top of that, physical activity can also help with depression and anxiety disorders, which affect a notable portion of the population. For people dealing with mental health challenges, this is *big* news.

Why do I consider exercise a 'magic' pill? Because medication often comes with serious side effects. Sure, you could injure yourself while exercising, but, overall, aerobic exercise has a pretty solid safety profile. However, with many medications, it's a different story. Gastrointestinal issues are some of the most common side effects of antidepressants, meaning people often feel bloated or experience nausea, vomiting, or diarrhea. Patients may also experience nutrient and electrolyte deficiencies, which can cause a host of other problems. For example, low sodium levels can cause hyponatremia, a known side effect of some antidepressants.[4] Hyponatremia, if left untreated, can lead to delirium, seizures, and even coma. Such side effects can have a negative influence on the brain, which isn't what you want when you're struggling with your mental health.

I'm not saying prescription medication doesn't have its place – it most certainly does – but most pills are far from magical. Exercise, on the other hand, is the closest intervention we have to a magic pill when it comes to improving our mental and physical health.

Running is *Almost* the Best Legal High (and the Most Fun You Can Have With Your Clothes On...)

When I came second in a 100-metre race in primary school, I experienced a high. It felt amazing. After completing my first ever City2Surf road race, I experienced an even more sustained high, even if it was mixed with feelings of exhaustion from the race and pain from severe shin splints.

Often referred to as 'runner's high', the experience is generally attributed to a burst of endorphins released during exercise. It's that feeling of total contentment that comes after a good run. To many, including myself, it's one of the best legal highs you can get.

During exercise, our bodies undergo a radical transformation that's unlike anything that occurs when we're sedentary or at rest. Our breathing becomes laboured and heavy, and our pulse speeds up as our heart works to transport much-needed oxygenated blood to our muscles. At the same time, endorphins act as analgesia to numb the pain in our muscles.

The runner's high feeling comes from the release of endocannabinoids – a chemical similar to what's found in cannabis – which cross the blood-brain barrier into the brain, where these neuromodulators cause brief psychoactive effects of calmness and reduced anxiety. Further, mice studies have found that the production of brain-derived neurotrophic factor (BDNF) is increased upon exercise, which promotes neurogenesis (production of new brain cells) in the hippocampus, an area of the brain linked to memory formation, resulting in less cognitive decline and improved brain performance.[5] What's more, human studies have demonstrated increases in hippocampal volume in regular exercisers, which is great news for those of us who are getting on in years, as the hippocampus shrinks with age, affecting memory and potentially leading to dementia.[6]

Not only does aerobic exercise get us high, but it also improves brain function in many different areas. So, it's time to put on those running shoes, start running towards a stronger, healthier mind, and have fun doing it.

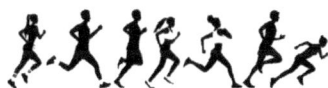

An Undeniable Success Rate

As a medical specialist in training, I had the opportunity to focus on obesity as an advanced endocrinology trainee in the renowned 'Metabolic Clinic', an intensive non-surgical weight management program in an Australian public hospital. The program consisted of a specialist medical team, nurse, physiotherapist or exercise physiologist, dietician, and psychologist, who met with each client on a regular basis for weigh-ins, anthropometric measures, such as waist circumference, and metabolic blood profiles, such as total cholesterol, LDL cholesterol, triglycerides, and uric acid levels. Clients also had sessions with relevant experts to discuss their motivations for overeating, which often included stress, comfort, and boredom. At the outpatient hospital gymnasium, clients also had access to an exercise program.

A 2021 study found that a multidisciplinary approach to weight management, such as the one used at the metabolic clinic, improved overall psychological health, including eating disorder symptoms.[7] During my work at the clinic, I observed similar results. The majority of clients enjoyed the positive experiences of the clinic, which led to improved compliance regarding diet and exercise. After they adopted healthier lifestyles, many of their health conditions improved to the extent that some people no longer required, or reduced, their medication. Some clients who were previously considered diabetic were even able to stop taking their insulin injections. Daily, I saw our multidisciplinary approach create positive change in people's lives.

However, at the clinic, there was still a subset of clients who were unable to effectively address their metabolic conditions. I knew this was an area of science and medicine where we could improve, so I began searching for answers, using myself as the first prospective lab rat.

Let It Burn! – Burning Fat, Getting Lean

Running burns calories at a rapid rate, which is great news for anyone who wants to shed a few kilos. Just 1 kilometre of running burns around 60 calories (or 1 mile burns approximately 100 calories), depending on weight, height, and running pace. While burning calories can translate to fat burning, not all running paces burn fat equally. It's time to talk about aerobic versus anaerobic running.

Aerobic – Lower-intensity runs (chatting comfortably pace). Heart rate remains under 65 percent of maximum, which means effort can be sustained for longer – think jogging or running a marathon. The body primarily uses oxygen and fat for fuel.

Anaerobic – Higher-intensity runs that use carbohydrates and lactic and amino acids for fuel. Oxygen and fat simply aren't sufficient fuel for shorter, more intense bursts of activity – think sprinting and hill runs.

I'll say it now: losing weight isn't the same as losing fat. Why? Because muscle weighs more than fat and is great for your health. Who doesn't want a little extra muscle? Fat, on the other hand, weighs less, and high amounts can lead to serious health problems. So, losing weight isn't ideal *if* you're losing muscle instead of fat. People can be light in weight and high in fat. Skinny people aren't necessarily healthier!

Clients often ask me, "How long should I run for to burn fat?" If you're doing a slow, low-intensity run, which uses fat for fuel but takes longer to burn calories, I recommend running longer than 30 minutes. I like to use the analogy that running is like igniting a candle. It takes effort to light a match and direct the flame to the top of the wick but once the candle is lit, osmosis transports the wax from the bottom to the top to ensure that the candle continuously burns bright. The key is to ensure that your candle is properly lit.

Interestingly, high-intensity exercise has also been shown to burn fat effectively via a different mechanism. After a bout of intense running, such as threshold or interval sprints, the total calorie consumption is higher. More calories are burned due to the intensity of the exercise and the demand on muscles and the cardiovascular system. But where does fat burning come in? During recovery, the body keeps consuming energy (burning calories), including fat stores, through a process called EPOC (excess post-exercise oxygen consumption).[8] That's right – runners can benefit from an afterburn effect that keeps the body burning fat *after* they've stopped running. Great news, right? Are you ready for some even better news? The afterburn effect can last for *hours* after you stop running. All you need to do is light the candle.

So, what happens when we pit high- and moderate-intensity running against each other? As we know, exercise at any intensity level does burn fat one way or another. However, one study found that HIIT (high-intensity interval training) was 28.5 percent more effective at reducing total absolute fat mass compared to moderate-intensity exercise.[9] Of course, exercise of any type is beneficial but if burning fat is your primary goal, it's time to up the intensity.

Generally, We Should Practise What We Preach

When I was the Fat Doc, I didn't always practise what I preached. Due to the nature of the medical specialist profession, patients and their carers often view us as gurus or oracles. In society, many people look up to us, seeing us as role models in various aspects of life.

Most healthcare professionals preach against unhealthy eating habits, smoking, and sedentary behaviour. We generally encourage our patients to live healthy lifestyles, which includes engaging in aerobic activities, such as running. However, behind closed doors, as the Fat Doc, my lifestyle was far from healthy, with obesity, high alcohol intake, poor dietary habits, and inadequate levels of physical activity all stacking up in one big pile of hypocrisy.

I've even heard stories of respiratory physicians in the 1960s doing their ward rounds, reviewing patients with emphysema, lung cancer, and tuberculosis, only to have a post-round cigarette afterwards. After all, smoking relieves stress, right? I'm sure there were many weak excuses they used to justify their actions. Back then, it wasn't uncommon to find doctors who smoked like chimneys – and this was well after the firm connection between smoking and lung cancer was established. Interestingly, even in the early 2000s, when I was a junior medical practitioner, I often saw nurses and doctors smoking during their breaks – and this still happens today. Stand outside any major public hospital, especially near a parking lot, and you'll see that the classic Aussie custom, the 'smoko', is alive and well.

As a medical specialist, I was guilty of the same hypocritical behaviour. Fast food, high-sugar sodas, persistent inactivity, and erratic sleep patterns were the norm for me. The problem is, it's also the norm for many other medical practitioners.

A study into the lifestyles of physicians discovered that only 10.8 percent of healthcare professionals consume fruits and vegetables in the recommended amounts. Shocked? Wait, it gets worse. Only 33 percent engage in moderate exercise three or more days per week, and over 80 percent consume alcohol regularly.[10] Do you think the lifestyles of the less healthy physicians in the study reflect what they teach their patients? Not by a long shot. Clearly, many physicians aren't practising what they preach. How can they effectively counsel their patients on healthy habits when they aren't following their own advice? Frankly, they can't.

When, as medical practitioners, we don't practise what we preach, we become less effective at facilitating positive change in our patients. It's as simple as that.

Birth of the 'Go Faster' Mentality

From six weeks old until age six, I was raised by my two grandmothers. Apparently, I wasn't feeding well – but can you blame me? It's pretty much expected when a baby is born several weeks premature. But because my mother had a strong Type A personality, everything had to be done on a schedule. If something disrupted her plans – like a fussy baby for instance – it became somebody else's problem. So, I was labelled a bad feeder, and my parents shuffled me off to live with my two grandmothers and an uncle. We were living in Hong Kong at the time.

I quite literally got a taste for competition early. At breakfast, my uncle and I would race each other eating our porridge. Ironically, it was English porridge. We thought it was the good stuff. My uncle and I would race every single day, but I could never beat him. "You must have a hole in your mouth," my grandmother would say. "You're always so slow. Why don't you go faster?" Good question. It's not like I was slacking off, but, no matter how hard I tried, I couldn't beat my uncle. I couldn't catch the person in front. I couldn't win. There, at the breakfast table, racing my uncle in a porridge eating competition, was where my 'go faster' mentality was born. When I started running, that same mentality fuelled me to outpace the competition, and it still does to this day. I'm always striving to go faster.

Run Doc Tips

The transformation from the Fat Doc to the Run Doc was inspired by the desire to live longer, free of disease after the birth of my third child and my daughter's success in cross-country. Find the biggest motivator to take the first step in *your* journey.

Running at low-intensity at least 30 minutes daily can assist in fat burning and weight maintenance.

When we, as clinicians, start practising what we preach, especially regarding running prescription, we'll be in a better position to combat the obesity epidemic.

"There is a superhero in all of us, we just need the courage to put on the cape."

– Superman

CHAPTER 2

═══════

RUN FOR YOUR MIND (SO YOUR MIND DOESN'T RUN YOU)

As a busy clinician, I found myself overworked. I was on call for multiple public and private hospitals; I was running three clinics weekly, and I provided specialist consultations at homes and aged care facilities.

I handled my on-call responsibilities with the utmost care, sleeping in a separate room from my partner whenever I was on call and prioritising work calls over family and friends at all times. After all, I was dealing with clients' lives, and missing a phone call could mean the difference between life and death. I took the Hippocratic oath seriously, but I was overcommitted, to the detriment of my own mental health (and physical health, too).

Due to chronic sleep deprivation and lack of physical exercise, I was stressed to the nth degree. I was snappy on the telephone, and, to those around me, I was unpleasant to deal with. I was abrupt. I was anxious each time the phone rang or displayed a hidden number, as it was likely a call from the hospital. I also experienced a pervasive mood of depression, especially during stressful discussions at work.

However, this all changed when I decided to transform into the Run Doc. Running literally saved my mental health and my life.

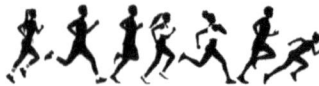

I Won't Say Running is a Mental Health Panacea, But...

As discussed earlier, the act of running, especially anything over 30 minutes, provides not only physical but also mental benefits through the secretion of endorphins (natural painkillers), serotonin (natural mood modulator), and endocannabinoids (responsible for runner's high).

Now, I don't want to say that running is a mental health panacea, but a massive 2023 *British Journal of Sports Medicine* review found that physical activity significantly improves symptoms of anxiety and depression.[11] Remember when I said running was a magic pill...? The authors of the study go on to suggest that exercise should be the foundational treatment for anxiety and depression – and I agree. As we know, the negative side effects of physical activity are practically negligible when compared to many medications. Whoever says you can't outrun your problems hasn't read the recent literature.

Running doesn't just improve our mental health but our mental fitness as well. One study showed that running improves reaction time and working memory in people with intellectual disabilities.[12] That's right – running can make you smarter.

Wait, it gets better. Regular exercise also reduces the risk of developing dementia and Alzheimer's disease.[13] That's why I highly recommend running for healthy ageing, from both a physical *and* mental standpoint.

Like me, those with mental health issues usually have coexisting medical conditions, such as metabolic syndrome, that would be amenable to physical activity. Really, once you understand how effective running is at treating such a wide range of issues, you can't help but wonder why we don't prescribe it more often.

Becoming a Doctor is Like Running an Ultramarathon

Growing up, I wanted to be a performer but once I got my medical degree, I realised I wanted to be a doctor more. Finally, I had the ability to really help people, which, to me, was a massive privilege. Once I graduated, I fell in love with what I was doing.

However, the life of an intern can be rough. Suddenly, I was the most junior person in the room, the smallest cog in the machine. It was a very depersonalising and difficult experience, largely because I was dealing with supervisors who had been through the same system as me. They had learnt in an environment where asking for help or showing emotion was considered a sign of weakness. Not all supervisors had this mentality – some were great – but some were, let's just say, typical.

When you're the smallest cog in the machine, you get stuck with many of the boring, menial tasks – and lots of them.

Your workload is *huge*. And if something goes wrong with the machine, who cops it? The smallest cog, of course. When something did go wrong, the newbies were always to blame, even if they had nothing to do with the incident.

On top of that, medical rotations were brutal. What do I mean? As medical interns, we usually got comfortable and efficient in our roles within three months. The problem was that every three months, we did a rotation, which meant we were thrust into different roles and had to start again. Just as we got comfortable with the terrain, they changed the landscape. For instance, we might start with a surgical term and just as we're getting comfortable, they pull us out and throw us into psychiatry. Before we know it, we're displaced again, landing in emergency medicine, and so on, and so on. With every rotation, our standing would reset. Suddenly, we were the junior members of the team again, and we were doing most of the dirty work. Of course, we also had middle managers (or registrars) bossing us around and sometimes taking credit for our work.

Unfortunately, all of this was a part of the medical culture and unlikely to change anytime soon, which was why a lot of people either completed a one-year internship and became general practitioners (GPs) or dropped out, whereas the rest of us stuck around and struggled our way through to the light at the end of the tunnel, seeking the holy grail of a specialist training qualification, through the arduous specialist training pathway. During this time, my mental health, happiness, and wellbeing took a massive hit, but running helped me get through it.

Although *being* a doctor is great, *becoming* a doctor is like running an ultramarathon. It's a rough undertaking. The first few months of an internship are like running a steep incline at the beginning of a race. You may have only run 3 kilometres, but it feels like thirty, and you're ready to quit. When you think about how much you've still got to go, the challenge before you seems impossible to overcome, which is why so many drop out as soon as they can. But I was determined to complete the race. Like in an ultramarathon, I just had to keep putting one foot in front of the other until I crossed the finish line.

How to Practise Mindfulness Meditation the Run Doc Way

Mindfulness involves staying connected to the 'now'. Through trial and error, I've developed a consistent routine that occasionally leads me to running nirvana (or running flow).

Running mindfully means zoning out in a positive way and involves three aspects:

1. **Focus on your breathing** – Concentrating on breathing is often recommended as the first step in many meditative practices. It can serve as an anchor to calm your mind and quiet your thoughts. When I first began to run, I used a simple 2:2 technique (two breaths in, and two breaths out). When I started my running routine, I could breathe deeply through my nose by relaxing my diaphragm and exhaling slowly. As I ran faster, I was able to watch my breathing without trying to control it.

2. **Define your why** – What's your reason for practising running meditation? It's helpful to establish an intention and come up with a statement that helps you stay focused on it. If the mind starts wandering during the run, repeating the intention usually helps bring it back to the present. My usual statement is a positive affirmation: "I get to run, and I can run strong, and I'm fully engaged with the present moment."

3. **Listen to your own breathing** – Although I now usually listen to podcasts while running (mainly about exercise and longevity), in the early days, I listened to music to dissociate from the often unpleasant experience of running – difficulty in breathing, painful feet and joints, and so on. Sometimes, I enjoy the

meditative experience of listening to the regularity of my breathing and the pitter-patter of my own feet striking different surfaces – pavement, sand, dirt roads, and even puddles of water or sloshy snow. Very occasionally, I engage into the flow state, which is like a microscopic but powerful dose of running nirvana. More on this in chapter eight.

Extreme Napping – Introducing the Nappuccino

I want to take a little detour here and introduce you to the nappuccino. What's that? It's exactly what it sounds like: combining a nap with caffeine. I know, I probably sound a little crazy right now – like I've had a few too many cappuccinos – but hear me out.

At around lunchtime, I like to have a short nap. By then, I've done my morning run, and a brief rest helps me recover. Before I take my nap, I drink a cup of coffee. Now, you're probably saying, "Jenson, coffee contains caffeine, and caffeine is a stimulant. Why would you take a stimulant right before a nap?" I'm glad you asked.

You see, timing is everything. After I drink my cup of coffee, I've got around ten minutes before the caffeine hits my system, which means I have ten minutes to fall asleep. If I miss that window, I'll be too overstimulated to sleep, as

I'm sure you can imagine. But if the timing is right, I'll wake up from a 20-minute nap with caffeine coursing through my veins, my energy levels through the roof. I could clean the house three times over, go for another run, or even write a book. I'm supercharged!

If the pressure of falling asleep before the caffeine kicks in is too much, the nappuccino may not be for you. It's a race you can't win with grit and determination. You have to relax and let the nap happen before you reach that caffeinated state.

Sometimes, I skip the nap altogether and just go for a run. What would you call combining coffee with running? Jogaccino?? Runoffee? Ruffee? I don't know. If you think of a good name, post it and tag me on social media. I would love to hear it.

Run Towards a Better Outlook on Life

When I started running again, within three months, I made several amazing discoveries. One, I had to buckle my belt at a new hole. Two, my shirts felt loose and oversized. Three, my double chin returned to a single one – a massive win! The little victories continued… One day, after a shower, I noticed that my love handles were shrinking and my one-pack was showing signs of becoming a sixpack, as the adipose tissue around my abdomen shrunk. A transformation was taking place before my eyes.

After each run, I felt a sense of accomplishment on multiple levels. My times were improving; I was running lighter; my arthritic knee pain was disappearing, and my shortness of breath was no longer rearing its ugly head. Further, my headaches were clearing up (likely due to less hypertensive episodes), and my sleep hygiene was improving. I was falling asleep quicker, slept through the night more often, and was feeling less tired during the day.

Unbeknownst to me, the rapid transformation from the Fat Doc to the Run Doc had begun.

Run Doc Tips

Running is as good if not better
than prescription medications
and psychological therapies for
treating mental health disorders.

Running is a form of mindfulness
meditation. It's empowering and
uplifting for your mind and soul.

Running is an effective way to
turn your one-pack into a sixpack
in the intermediate term.

"GUY: 'Well, yah see Doc, the problem is obesity runs in my family.'

DOC: 'No, the problem is *nobody* runs in your family.'"

– Anonymous

CHAPTER 3

THE ELIXIR OF YOUTH STARTS AT YOUR FEET

Some say that being healthy is the mere absence of disease. But after more than two decades of clinical practice, helping over 10,000 patients, I've learnt there's a certain group of people who are stuck in the subhealth state. They're not quite diseased – that is, they don't have full-blown diabetes or anything of that nature – but they're showing early warning signs that something is wrong. For example, they might have mild fatty liver disease, narrowing of the coronary arteries, or slightly elevated triglycerides. It's common for such clients to walk into my office with vague symptoms, such as poor concentration, daytime drowsiness, aches, indigestion, nervousness, and reduced exercise tolerance, wanting to know why they seem to be stuck in this purgatorial state between health and disease.

In this subset of clients, I've found that, in many instances, a daily dose of running (more than 20 minutes in duration) to achieve a heart rate in the maximum aerobic function (MAF) zone provides a kickstart to reversing the chronic inflammation of subhealth and moves people towards healthy ageing and longevity.[14]

When it comes to the elixir of youth, there are no shortcuts. If you want to age with health and vitality on your side, you must do the work. The elixir of youth starts at your feet.

When Was the Last Time You Went to Your Doctor for a Chat?

Our medical system works in a way in which no news is generally good news. If you don't hear from your doctor, everything is probably fine. In Western culture, we operate under the assumption that we should only visit our doctors when something is wrong. We wait for the disease to strike before we act, whereas we could be focusing on prevention first.

Often, people come to me for a chat. They're not necessarily suffering from any ailments, but they want to take a preventative approach. While these interactions resemble casual chats, that's just a front, a masquerade. During the consultation, I'm performing a physical and mental health check and recommending primary prevention measures.

After these chats, my patients leave a lot happier, even though I haven't prescribed any medication or performed any surgery – and I don't need to. It's amazing how many health issues that would normally be medicated can be solved or alleviated with the right prescription of diet and exercise. Sure, we can prescribe a pill for almost any ailment these days, but most medication comes with side effects, some of them quite severe. If a bit of healthy eating and regular exercise might be the solution, isn't it worth exploring first? And if running or the like doesn't solve the problem, we can always reach for the prescription pad when it's needed.

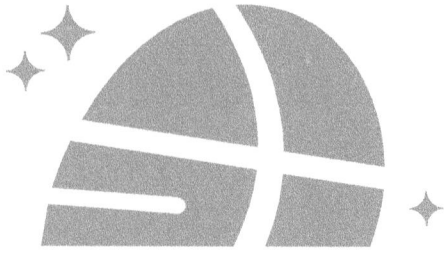

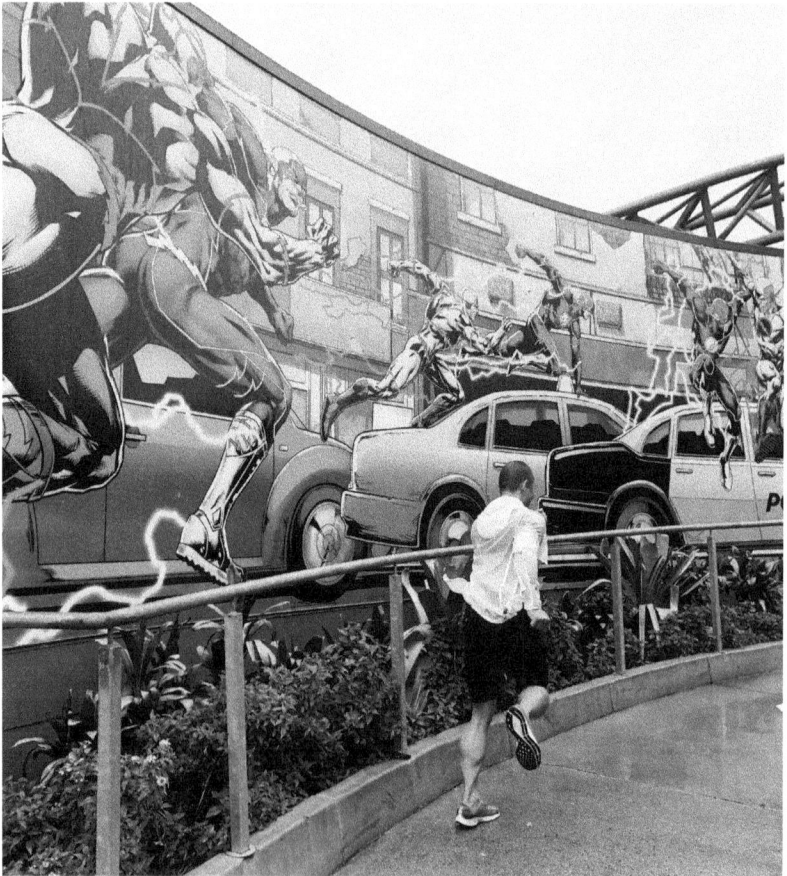

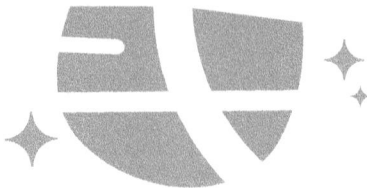

Outpace ageing.
Running towards longevity.

Outpace Ageing, Run Towards Longevity

As a healthy ageing specialist, I'm often requested to give expert medical advice for secondary prevention associated with the ageing process, for example, after a stroke, heart attack, or hip fracture. While I happily offer advice wherever I can, I find it even more rewarding and enjoyable to identify modifiable risk factors in the middle-aged (35-plus) population that can be amenable to natural interventions, such as running and healthy eating.

When prescribing exercise, I often quote the Aerobics Center longitudinal study undertaken by Lee and colleagues, which examined 14,345 men with a mean age of 44 years. The study found that during a follow-up of 11.4 years, every improvement of 1-MET (metabolic equivalent) lowered all-cause and CVD (cardiovascular disease) mortality by 15 percent for participants with "stable fitness" and 19 percent for those with "fitness gain."[15] Therefore, simply maintaining a good fitness level is enough to boost your life expectancy, and improving your fitness comes with even greater benefits. To further highlight the power of aerobic exercise, a follow-up study found that running for only 5–10 minutes per day at slow speeds (under 10 km/h) was enough to significantly reduce all-cause and CVD mortality.[16] Studies repeatedly show that running wards off stroke and heart disease, and reduces your risk of death, period. So, if you want to live a long and healthy life, running may be the elixir of youth you've been looking for.

My Grandmother's Secret to Warding Off Dementia

I have no qualms about admitting to my clients that my maternal grandmother was diagnosed with dementia at age 86. Then I tell them she's still alive at 94, walking without a stick and looking like a fit 80-year-old. Both her younger and older sister also suffered from dementia, which presented in their late-60s and mid-70s respectively, but my grandmother was well into her 80s when she was diagnosed.

What's her secret? She regularly exercised, walking 6–8 km daily, including up and down stairs, to the local markets for her groceries.

In 2008, a randomised control study of 138 people with mild cognitive impairment (mild forgetfulness, not full-blown dementia) demonstrated that a six-month program of regular exercise improved certain aspects of memory over 18 months.[17] Essentially, the literature provides a possible explanation for how my grandmother outlived her two sisters and is still happily walking around at 95.

Want Great Skin? Here's the Trick

So many people spend thousands, often tens of thousands, of dollars in their lifetimes on expensive skincare products – facials, botox, plastic surgeries, to name a few. Did you know that running can help you achieve similar effects (without the high cost and potential side effects)?

When we run, we boost blood circulation to our skin, causing our pores to open. This circulation boost increases oxygen and nutrient delivery, which is what gives us an immediate post-exercise glow. Enhanced blood flow also helps skin cells regenerate and remove toxins more efficiently, while also decreasing our levels of the stress hormone cortisol. Running and its stress-lowering effects are also beneficial for treating chronic skin conditions like eczema and acne.[18]

For many of us, great skin is only a run away.

The Key to Unbreakable Bones

Osteoporosis is marked by gradual bone loss and can lead to serious complications, such as hip fractures, leading to significant morbidity and even death. Fractures mainly occur from traumatic injuries in the young and middle-aged, while falls are the main causes in the older age group.

Being a weight-bearing exercise, running reduces the rate of bone loss and conserves bone tissue, lowering the risk of fractures. Additionally, a systematic review of 116 studies, involving 25,160 participants, found that balance and functional exercise, such as running, reduce the risk of falling by 24 percent.[19]

As we age, running or another form of functional exercise is practically mandatory if we want to conserve bone density and avoid fall-related injuries.

Who Says Running is Bad for Your Joints?

As the Fat Doc, I regularly felt a gnawing pain in my knees, especially when I stood or sat for more than half an hour, walked up and down stairs, or attempted to jog for a few metres. At the very least, I had moderate knee osteoarthritis (or degenerative joint disease). No doubt, my increased weight contributed to the extra stressors on my cartilage.

After I shed around 20 kg over three months, my joint pain all but disappeared. Seven years later, I compared my most recent knee X-ray (radiograph) to the one from my Fat Doc days – and guess what? My knees had notably improved. The space between my femur (thigh bone) and tibia (shin bone) is now slightly wider, despite all the running mileage. But isn't running supposed to be bad for our joints? Let's bust that myth right now.

Mounting evidence suggests that running *doesn't* cause osteoarthritis or any other joint disease. A 2017 study found that recreational runners had lower rates of hip and knee osteoarthritis (3.5 percent) compared to competitive runners (13.3 percent) and non-runners (10.2 percent).[20] According to a 2018 study, the rate of hip and knee arthritis among 675 marathon runners was approximately half the rate expected within the general US population.[21] Further, a 2022 analysis of 24 studies found no evidence of significant harm to the cartilage lining the knee joints on MRIs taken just after running.[22] A large meta-analysis of 15 studies even suggests running has a protective effect on the joints, decreasing the possibility of ever needing knee joint surgery.[23]

In my case, running saved my life. Not only that, but it reversed the signs of ageing and cured my knee osteoarthritis to the extent that I no longer suffer from knee pain.

Ken's Dodgy Back

My good running friend, Dr Ken, developed a lumbar disc injury from lifting moderate weights in a seated position between client telephone consults. When he returned to running, the lower back pain and sciatica would appear within several kilometres, which, unsurprisingly, affected his performance. To add salt to his injury, he was also nursing a moderate-severe ankle sprain that he sustained during com-petition several years before.

When he asked me to help him recover from his back injury and return to trail running, I was a seasoned road mar-athoner but not yet a trail runner. His trust in me as a trail running coach led me to complete my first Six-Foot Track Trail Ultramarathon and eventually attain a Level 3 Trail and Ultramarathon High Performance Coaching accreditation with Athletics Australia. This led to completing the Ultra-Trail Australia 100 km (UTA100) and successfully qualifying and being chosen to participate in the 2023 Ultra-Trail du Mont Blanc (UTMB), the holy grail of trail running – or the running equivalent of the Tour de France!

In return, I was able to share with Ken some of my lower back remedy exercises, which helped him to later successes. He was able to complete the 2023 UTA50 race in a respectable time that he was happy with, pain-free.

Let's Talk Recovery

Many people believe that a runner's improvement occurs during a tough workout, but, in fact, it actually happens during recovery. That's right – improvement and adaptation occur in the immediate period after a workout, for example, with recovery fuelling, and in the intermediate period, for example, with nappuccinos and sleep.

A crucial pillar of rapid recovery is the 80/20 running rule, which dictates that roughly 80 percent of our training should be done at low intensity (MAF pace) and the remaining 20 percent at moderate- or high-intensity. The beauty of this training process is that we sustain very few overuse injuries and recover from acute running injuries quicker. If you're unsure how hard to train, I recommend giving the 80/20 method a try.

Skinny Doesn't = Healthy (a Cautionary Tale)

Dr A was a medical practitioner whom I respected and looked up to. Previously, we worked together in one of the medical centres I attended weekly, and I knew him as a gentle soul. He was in his late-40s, slim, married with no children, and regularly walked his dog. Sounds healthy enough, right? To the eye, Dr A was a healthy guy.

However, after experiencing chest pains and dialling for help, he was found unresponsive in his own office. The likely cause of death was a heart attack. The thing is, Dr A hadn't exhibited any cardiovascular warning symptoms, making him a sad reminder of the importance of middle-aged health professionals regularly reviewing their cardiovascular health. Not only that, but we should all be engaging in moderate cardio exercise, such as running, on a regular basis to keep our cardiovascular systems healthy. There are very few con-traindications when it comes to running.

For first-time runners, a good screening questionnaire is the APSS (adult pre-exercise screening system) from ESSA

(Exercise & Sports Science Australia), which you can find online.[24] If you have any medical conditions or injuries, the test can help you determine the level of exercise you can safely handle.

Both Dr A and my uncle experienced unexpected heart attacks in their 40s, practically in the prime of their lives. Sometimes, we really don't see a heart attack coming until it's too late, which is why we need to be proactive in both preventing and diagnosing any issues.

Unfortunately, caregivers may be particularly susceptible to cardiovascular disease, with a systematic review finding that carers who provided intense caregiving (over nine hours of informal care per week) to ill or disabled individuals were more likely to suffer cardiovascular disease than non-caregivers.[25] Indeed, I wouldn't be doing my duty as a medical practitioner if I didn't do my best to try to save the lives of other carers and clinicians by shining a light on the problem.

Dr A's passing was a central inspiration for this book. When one of our own – one who served his local community and should have served for many more years – is taken away from us by sudden coronary artery disease, it's high time to discuss the very important issue of our own health, because awareness saves lives.

You're Never Too Old to Run

When I approach middle-aged or older clients about starting to run, I usually receive one of several common responses: "I'm too old to run because…"

"…It could worsen my arthritis."

"…I could fall over."

"…Nobody my age runs."

It's time to talk about Ed Whitlock.

At 85 years old, the late Ed Whitlock set a long-distance running record by completing the Toronto Waterfront Marathon in 3 hours 56 minutes 34 seconds, becoming the oldest person to run a 26.2-mile (42.2-km) marathon in under four hours.

According to a *New York Times* article, Ed "… raced in 15-year-old shoes and a singlet that was 20 or 30 years old. He has no coach. He follows no special diet. He does not chart his mileage. He wears no heart-rate monitor. He takes no ice baths, gets no massages. He shovels snow in the winter and gardens in the summer but lifts no weights, does no situps or push-ups. He avoids stretching, except the day of a race. He takes no medication, only a supplement that may or may not help his knees."[26]

He's the ideal example of what healthy ageing can look like, and he's someone I make a point to mention to my older clients who are hesitant to start running. Although Ed died of prostate cancer at age 86, he lived a full life, running marathons and breaking records well into his final years.

I share these lessons from Ed Whitlock's running career with clients:

- Aiming for a strong running peak in middle-age is important.

- It's possible to have a reasonable level of fitness (including running marathons in your 80s) through regular training.

- Running after 65 is possible and can improve your overall functionality and even prolong life by increasing bone density and muscle strength through repetitive weight bearing. It helps with fall prevention and improves lung capacity, cardiovascular function, and memory, and makes you a happier and less stressed human being.

Run Doc Tips

1

Running helps your body turn off the damaging chronic inflammatory state and reverse the ageing process.

2

Running is beneficial for your skin, joints, heart, lungs, and mind.

3

I highly recommend the 80/20 training method for running.

"Money is cheap.
Time is priceless!"

– The Run Doc

CHAPTER 4

YOU'RE BORN TO RUN

As I gradually transitioned from the Fat Doc to the Run Doc, I spent many hours observing how my daughter (who would later become junior school cross-country captain) trained. I also observed how my infant son effortlessly ran while at play – smiling, carefree, barefoot, arms and legs moving in an efficient way, and, most importantly, relaxed. It was very similar to how his oldest sister ran *with* training.

When I first discovered the joys of barefoot running, I realised that my lap times at the Bert Oldfield dog park were almost equivalent to when I wore running shoes. In fact, I was able to run faster for longer due to a lower rate of perceived effort (RPE) and average heart rate. With better running biomechanics (better foot strike and shorter foot contact time), my body was expending less energy for the same distance.

We are indeed born to run!

Going Slow Was Never an Option (Born to Run)

When we moved to Australia, I took on a lot of responsibilities within the family. One of those responsibilities was navigation. Before my parents got really busy with establishing and running a business, we went on several road trips every school holidays and sometimes even on weekends. Dad would drive, and I would navigate from the front passenger seat. Back then, there were no smartphones or navigation apps, so I had to do it the old-fashioned way: by reading paper maps.

At 7 years old, I was burdened with the heavy responsibility of guiding us to our destination, which I didn't always do without making at least a few mistakes. When I did mess up, I copped Dad's wrath. But even though I made mistakes, my navigation skills were pretty good, and Dad saw this and nurtured those skills (in his own way). On long trips, Mum and my brother would be in the back, snoring, but I wasn't allowed to sleep because I had a job to do. Occasionally, I was able to persuade Dad to let me have a five-minute nap, but that was it. The navigator's job never ends. When your parents have such high expectations of you, you're forced to grow up fast.

At one point, Mum and Dad were both working eight hours per day, so my younger brother and I had to fend for ourselves. Because I was the eldest, naturally, a lot of the responsibility fell on me, including making sure we were fed. We always had food in the fridge, but my parents never taught me how to cook. Their expectations of me were so high that they figured I had seen them cook frequently enough to know what to do, so I was forced to wing it and learn on the job. *How hard could it be to use the rice cooker? Frying an egg, that looks easy. Steak? I guess you just cook it until there's no blood.* So, at age 8, I was cooking gourmet fried rice for the whole family.

My parents weren't being cruel by putting so much responsibility on my shoulders. In a way, they were nurturing me. They knew I was capable, and they knew I could handle the responsibility. I'm not saying it's the right approach for everyone – some kids need to be nurtured differently – but being pushed to learn, grow, and become independent at such a young age prepared me for many of life's later challenges. Incidentally, this experience scarred me for most of my teenage years, and my culinary skills temporarily peaked at age 8. I didn't improve at all until I turned 18.

Shoes are Overrated

It's important for runners, especially beginners, to run barefoot over soft grass. When we consider which muscles we use while running, the large muscles of the lower limbs often come to mind: the calves, hamstrings, and quads. However, the intrinsic (or the small) muscles of the feet are equally important, as they help to stabilise and modulate each foot during the heel strike and toe off in conjunction with the larger muscles. Essentially, these muscles modulate the ground contact force of each foot, which indirectly relates to running efficiency and overuse injuries.

One study focusing on 60 young adults found that an eight-week barefoot running program "increased foot strike index and reduced ground-reaction force and loading rates" for runners who were previously shod, suggesting the potential for injury prevention.[27]

In many ways, maximalist or super shoes attenuate the proprioception and intrinsic muscle strength response in the foot, which can adversely affect performance if worn too often. By practising jogging or sprinting on the grass with 'naked feet', we increase the strength of the intrinsic muscles and develop a better appreciation of the part they play in running.

Sometimes Nature Knows Best

The endurance running theory proposes that humans' ability to run long distances in a sustainable way shaped the course of our evolution by providing us the possibility to hunt. Most large mammals easily outrun humans during short bursts of running (sprints), but none can match our pace for longer than a few minutes. By chasing animals over distances without a break, humans forced their prey to overheat and collapse or at least slow their pace and weaken enough to be killed swiftly. The practice of running an animal to death, formally known as 'persistence hunting', brought a steady supply of nutrient-rich meat into the early hunter-gatherer diet.

Biologically, the persistence hunting and 'born to run' theories of human evolution make sense because we've developed physical attributes required to be good endurance runners. The Achilles tendon, which connects the calf muscles (plantar flexors) and heel acts as a spring mechanism, storing and releasing energy. Notably, this tendon is absent in other species of great apes that can walk but not run. Humans are much more adept at sweating due to having very little fur on their bodies and a dense concentration of sweat glands in the skin – several hundred for every square centimetre. Therefore, we're able to adapt to heat more efficiently than most of the prey we chase. Additionally, we can both mouth and nose breathe, which is important when running.

Clearly, running is as natural to us as breathing, seeing, and hearing, and to live a sedentary lifestyle by choice goes against millions of years of human evolution. You *were* born to run!

I'd Like to Say I Finish Every Race But... (How to Prevent DNFs)

While we're born to run, it doesn't mean running is always easy. I'm no quitter, but, as much as it pains me to admit, I have dropped out of two races in the past. The first was due to physical reasons; the second was more mental.

Dropout number one occurred during the Treble Buster at Forster. I was pacing my colleague and friend, Ken, who later became my running student. We were supposed to be completing a half marathon, but I had to DNF (did not finish) at 10 kilometres because I was cramping all over. I had run a tough race (Six Foot Trail Ultramarathon) ten days before and was in no condition to be running hard again. Dropping out was tough for me, but I had run out of juice, and I couldn't physically keep going.

DNF number two was, interestingly, another Treble. I was dehydrated and overheating, but the physical issues weren't what did me in, although they did contribute to my troubles. Basically, my brain wasn't in the game, and I was overthinking things too much. It was a circuit race, and, on the second of six laps, I mentally malfunctioned and couldn't keep going. Again, dropping out was tough for me, but, at the time, it was what I felt like I had to do. It's okay to quit sometimes, but don't make it a habit. To this day, after 40 marathons, I haven't had another DNF. Let's hope it stays that way!

When running a tough race, it's important to have multiple goals. Goal A might be to get a PB (personal best). If you can't meet goal A, goal B might be to finish the race. If goal B is out of reach, you might even have a goal C, and so on. Yes, we want to finish every race we enter, but it's not always possible, which is why having backup goals is important. If I'm struggling in a race, I think, *Jenson, you chose to run. You signed up, you paid the money, and you showed up on race day. Think of the above knee amputee, the guy with emphysema carrying an oxygen tank on his back, and the mother pushing two kids in a pram. You've got it easier than them – so finish the race!*

For me, running is a privilege, and remembering this keeps me going whenever a race gets tough.

Born to Run 'Naked'

Once I discovered that a weekly or fortnightly 'naked' (feet) run improved my running form, I began prescribing this to some of my clients, especially those with foot issues – metatarsalgia, Achilles tendinopathy, plantar fasciitis, and other causes of foot pain.

My method consists of sprinting the length of a soccer field and jogging the width, repeating 4–10 times, depending on the runner's ability.

Counterintuitively, running naked actually promotes some characteristics of optimal running form:

1. Promotes forefoot to midfoot landing and discourages heel striking.

2. Improves body posture.

3. Optimises running cadence (approximately 180 strides per minute).

4. Improves the proprioceptive abilities of the sole.

If you're looking to improve your running form, running naked is the key.

Run Doc Tips

1

Sometimes taking on a seemingly mammoth task brings out your best self and instigates the growth process.

2

Running is a privilege. When it doesn't go well, try to look for a key positive learning from each challenging running experience.

3

Running 'naked' can help develop better sole proprioception with the ground and, in turn, improve running dynamics with shoes.

"Explore your pain cave,
then expand it, and
embrace the suffering
during the race."

– The Run Doc

CHAPTER 5

FREEDOM IS YOURS

As I continued to morph from the Fat Doc into the Run Doc, I had the revelation that running could provide unlimited freedom, no matter the circumstances.

In my life, I had been so constrained by an overcommitment to work, study, and research that I didn't allocate sufficient time to relaxation and, most of all, recovery. However, attaining level three, high-performance, ultra and trail running coach status gave me specific insights into how to boost the performance of my athletes, including adequate training stimulus and sufficient recovery to allow adaptation of the mind and body to occur. Of course, I also needed to make adjustments to my own training and allow proper recovery time.

When I bumped into Dr G (a 65-year-old radiologist who completed the Ultra-Trail Mt. Fuji three times) at the 2022 Ultra-Trail Australia (UTA) 100 kilometres, he aptly summed up the freedom of running: "When I go out running, I don't take my pager, I don't even take my phone. I wear my CASIO watch. I don't want to be contacted. This is my *me* time."

For many of us, running has the potential to deliver ultimate freedom in our busy lives.

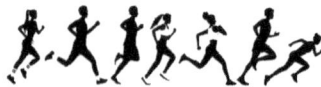

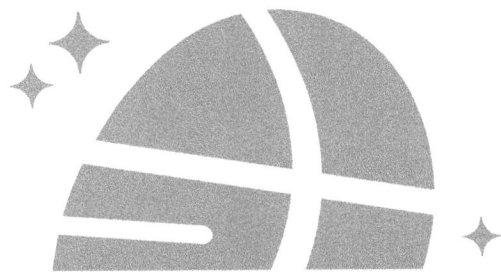

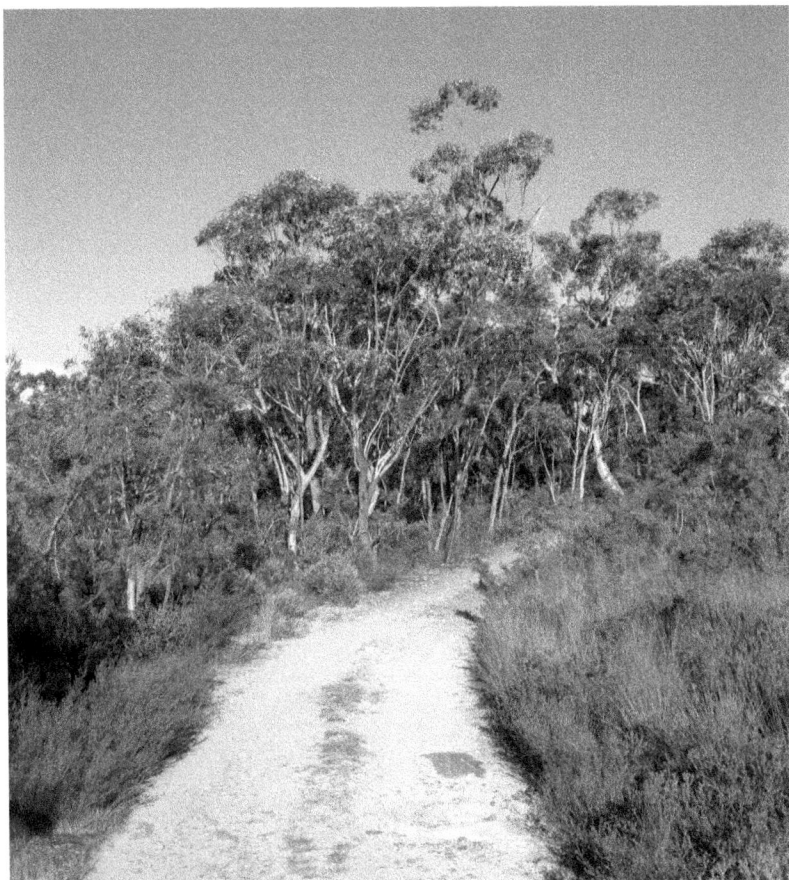

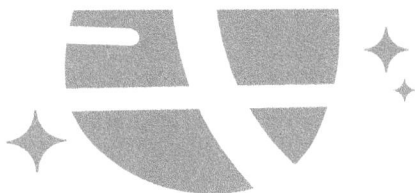

Discover the ultimate freedom through running.

Running is the Ultimate Freedom

How does Dr G achieve ultimate freedom through running? While running, he's able to choose his route, both start and finish as well as signposts along the way. He's able to choose when and how he runs, with his choice of form and breathing pattern. He's able to accessorise with his CASIO watch, shoes, socks, arm warmers, headwear, *everything*. He can choose to run with a phone, headlamp, running poles – the possibilities are endless!

With so many controllable variables, who wouldn't want to run? After all, most of us have financial, spiritual, work, family, vocational, and other commitments that are often time-consuming and sometimes uninspiring and mundane. Running provides an opportunity to temporarily escape the realities of life *and* experience feelings of euphoria as well as a sense of achievement, because you *are* achieving something!

The positive effects of running continue to multiply. As discussed earlier, not only does running improve our physical wellbeing and help ward off harmful disease, but it also reduces the risk of falls and other accidents and, of course, improves our mental health. By enhancing our cognition, we also enhance other aspects of our lives, including our ability to function at work and at home.

So, for the small cost of 20 minutes minimum (on the treadmill or outside) per day, we receive at least a threefold return on our time investment through improved productivity and performance, *and* we get to experience ultimate freedom. What's not to love about running?

Running is an Endless Adventure – Anything Can Happen!

At the time of writing, I've completed 40 marathons, including road, trail, and ultramarathons, over four continents. No two marathons are ever the same, even on the same course, as conditions can differ so much from day to day. Weather, including temperature and humidity, road or trail surface, other runners, other people on the course, your own nutrition, sleep, and other pre-race habits can all influence your results and overall experience on race day.

The unpredictability of the marathon also augurs well for the optimists among us, as, generally, the race doesn't truly begin until the 32-kilometre (20-mile) mark, and tiny adjustments to your approach and mindset at any time can improve race dynamics and performance. For example, in the 2023 London Marathon, I hit a very good patch in the first 5 kilometres and ran my fastest ever half-marathon distance. After struggling with cramps at the 25 km mark, I decided to utilise the Jeff Galloway 'run-walk' method for the remainder of the race. I felt so good that I sprinted the final mile (past Big Ben) all the way to the finish line to score my fastest marathon time to date!

Running Shapes Your Personality – for the Better!

My philosophy is that running can improve some parts of our personalities. When we run, we become much more organised in our work-life balance, living in the now and being mindful of every moment. Indeed, as a highlight, running has helped me find the gift in suffering. Handling being the sole breadwinner of the family and weathering the storm during the COVID-19 pandemic, especially homeschooling my three children and balancing work re-sponsibilities, were only possible through the learnings of my regular running routines.

On a physiological level, the changes that occur at heart rate zones 2–4 (65–88 percent of max heart rate) mimic the sometimes abnormal responses triggered by the sympathetic nervous system (flight or fight response) during bouts of anger and anxiety, as well as situations that elicit stress. By learning to control breathing during periods of zone two running, you can adopt a similar strategy at other times during the stress response to help de-escalate a situation.

Additionally, learning to complete each workout and finish every marathon teaches the mind and body resilience as well as mental toughness, which are essential to surviving and thriving in today's world and beyond. For example, if I sprain an ankle during a trail marathon, I don't just pull out of the race. Instead, I devise a strategy to improve my chances of completing the marathon. I might, for instance, use racing poles to off-load the weight on the affected ankle.

Practising resilience while running translates to building resilience in life.

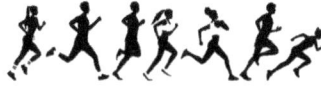

Create the Freedom to Run

Running is also a great way to nurture the mind. Essential to the 'central governor' theory, proposed by South African scientist Tim Noakes, are the concepts of peripheral and central fatigue.[28]

Peripheral fatigue is when the muscle itself is the cause of fatigue. For example, when you're running, your quads begin to 'burn' and fatigue due to a build-up of acidity that, in turn, slows you down, potentially bringing you to a stop. However, the central governor model opposes the idea of peripheral fatigue, stating that it's not the muscles that cause fatigue, but the brain.

As the brain is the body's central control room, training it can improve performance in individuals, even if their physiology remains the same. For example, world-class runner and men's marathon record holder, Eliud Kipchoge, has similar

VO2 max (maximum oxygen consumption) to some of his fellow competitors, yet he often beats their times by several minutes through his mental toughness. Kipchoge once remarked, "Athletics is not so much about the legs. It's about the heart and mind." He also stated, "Only the disciplined ones in life are free. If you are undisciplined, you are a slave to your moods. You are a slave to your passions. That's a fact."[29] Eliud Kipchoge is a shining example of how consistently training the mind can positively impact the running body.

Freedom to Challenge Your Mind (Visit Your Pain Cave)

I support the notion that completing most endurance events (longer than 1.5 km) is 90 percent mental and only 10 percent physical. In fact, my own ultramarathon experiences lead me to believe this ratio may be even higher. During training, I often challenge myself to complete several variations of a running workout, which leads me to the 'pain cave':

1. Progressive 1-km repeats: One method that improves my mental toughness is completing progressive repetitions of a set distance, for example, 1-kilometre or 1-mile repeats, starting at a comfortable pace and finishing at threshold pace.

2. Progressive 1-km repeats (variation): Another method for mental toughness is ten repeats. First repeat is a warm-up. The next three repeats are at slower than half-marathon pace (HMP). The next three repeats are at marathon pace. The final three repeats are at faster than HMP.

    Metaphorically, I see the warm-up as an actual warm-up, the first 3 km as running towards the entrance to the pain cave, the next 3 km as entering and reaching the cavernous part of the cave, and the final 3 km as grabbing a shovel and digging my way out of the cave.

I find the act of completing these workouts – or finding my pain cave and exploring it – to be one of the most effective ways to simulate the experience of reaching a difficult point in a race.

2023 Glow Worm Tunnel Marathon: A Great Case Study for Exercising My Freedom to Explore My Pain Cave

Running frees your mind to explore the darkest and most challenging parts of your pain cave – which is exactly what I did during the 2023 Glow Worm Tunnel Marathon

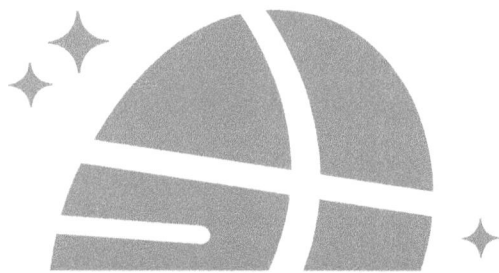

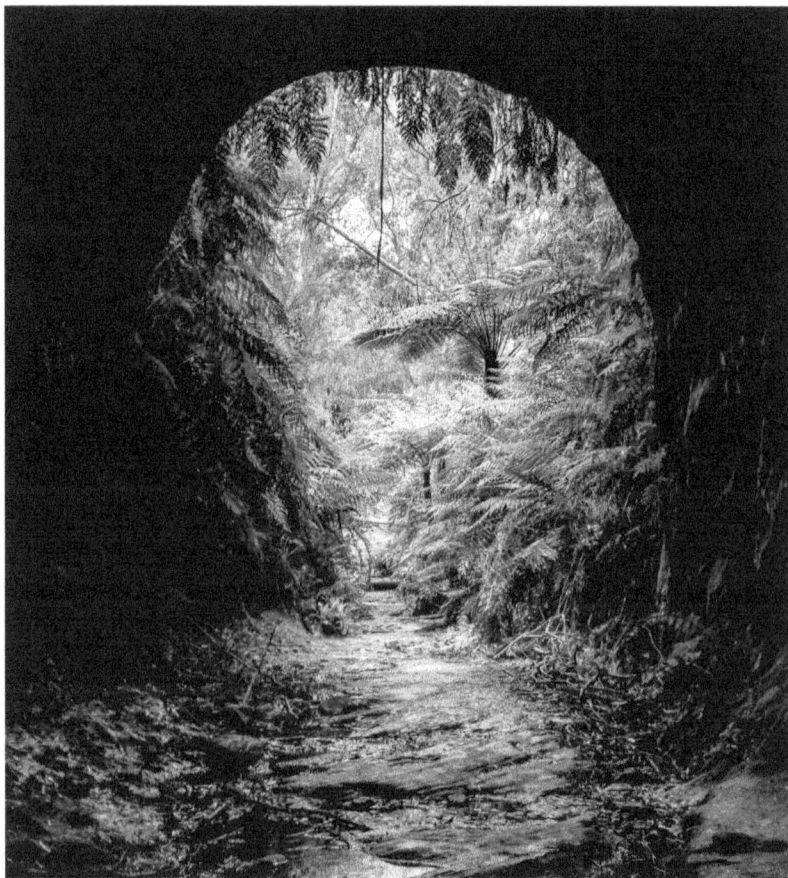

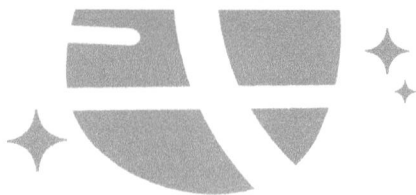

Glow Worm Tunnel,
Wollemi National Park,
NSW Australia.

(43 kilometres with 1600-metre elevation). In that race, I improved my personal best by 72 minutes and attained sixth place in my age group.

The highlights of that race were:

1. Below 0°C morning prep. Both my front and rear windscreens had frosted over, making the journey to the start line impossible until I had defrosted the ice.

2. Three significant climbs ranging 350–550 metres in elevation (total elevation 1600 metres), but the magnitude of incline during ascent was often greater than 15 percent.

3. An out and back 500-m x 2 (1000-m) tunnel traverse in darkness, with rough terrain and two river crossings.

Essentially, a B race is a good dress rehearsal for an A race. For example, the weather extremes (from below zero to 25°C), the extremes of the inclines, and the spacing of aid stations were very similar to the UTMB course.

After the 2022 race, I remarked on my Facebook blog, "Determination and grit … is when your mind is telling you to shut down, and the heart is urging you to push on and fight till the end!"

At this time, I was working on expanding my pain cave, which included:

1. Specific elevation work, such as regular long hill repeats (up to 900 metres).

2. Regular progressive 1-km repeats and 1-km variation repeats (as discussed earlier).

3. The use of poles on steep inclines, which off-loaded my lower limb muscles on climbs.

4. Completion of specific trail ultramarathon races (2022 Ultra-Trail Australia UTA100, 2023 Six Foot Track Marathon, 2023 Ultra-Trail Australia UTA50).

By regularly exploring, expanding, and embracing my pain cave, I've exercised my freedom to run and, in doing this, made significant gains in my trail running capacity over a 12-month period. By constantly exercising freedom to expand their pain caves, runners can not only improve their physical endurance but also their mental capacity, expanding their horizons and strengthening the mind-body-heart connection.

Run Doc Tips

Running provides a great opportunity to escape the realities of life and grants you the ultimate freedom (of choice).

Running a marathon is the ultimate test of endurance and an expression of your freedom!

Running workouts give you the opportunity to exercise your body as well as your mind, especially when you discover and expand your 'pain cave'.

"Don't let your age
control your life.
Let your life control
your age."

– Anthony Douglas Williams

CHAPTER 6

RUNNING IS FOR EVERYONE

Dick Hoyt first pushed his son, Rick, who is quadriplegic and has cerebral palsy, in a specialized wheelchair in the Boston Marathon in 1980. Over their running careers, Dick and Rick completed 32 Boston Marathons together!

Seeing video footage of Dick exhibiting superhuman physical and mental resilience and Rick encouraging his father to strive for his best evokes strong emotions. Rick, living vicariously through his father's feats of endurance, is both a physical burden and a mental inspiration. Together, they inspired countless others who might be in similar situations.

After the first race, Rick said to his father, "Dad, when I'm running, it feels like I'm not handicapped."[30] Ultimately, Team Hoyt proved to the world that running *is* for everyone.

Why I Can't Run Like Most People

When I did cross-country in high school, I loved the camaraderie. Every year, we would compete in the City2Surf race, which was a 14-kilometre run, wearing our school singlets. We were a team, and I was proud to represent the school.

Unfortunately, I still hadn't learnt how to properly run a long-distance race. I would run hard for the first 8 kilometres or so until I hit Heartbreak Hill, at which point terrible shin splints would almost bring me to a stop. Because I always had a good first split, people often questioned what had happened.

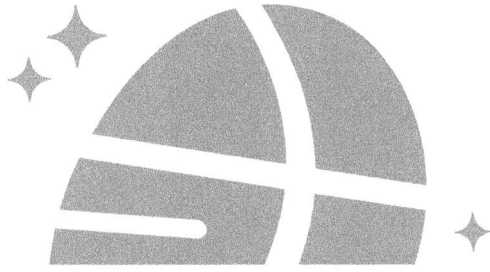

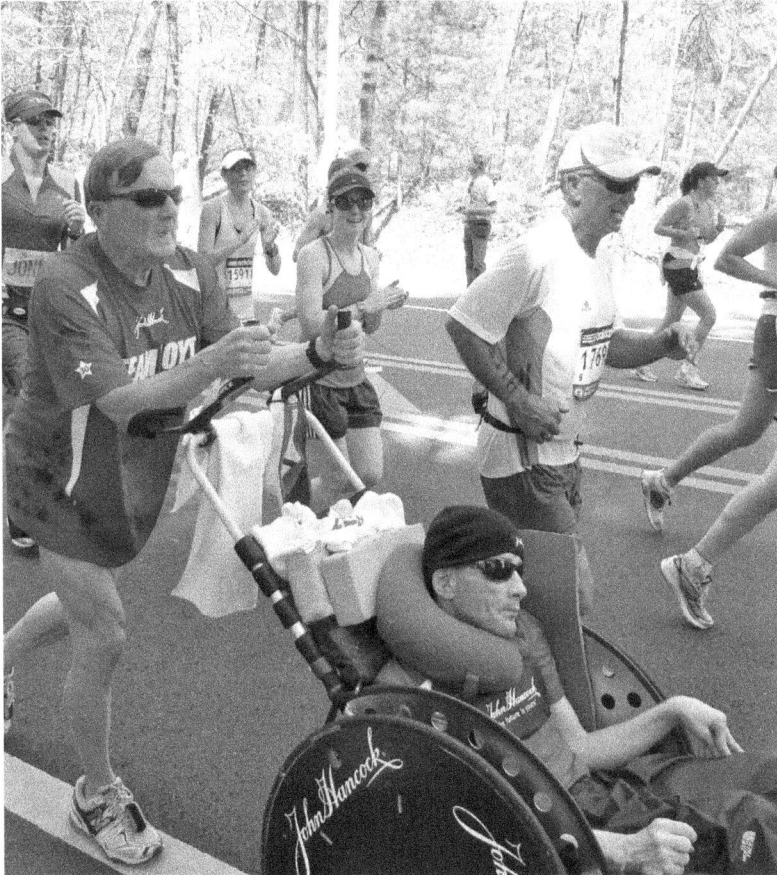

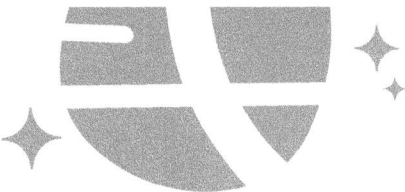

Team Hoyt in Wellesley.[31]

"Why were you so slow?"

"Were you injured?"

"Did someone else run the last half of the race for you?"

All I could say was that I did my best.

Later, I learnt that a physical condition, along with my questionable 'go hard early' strategy, was affecting my ability to run comfortably. I was born with bilateral genu valgum and recurvatum, which means I'm bow-legged. Later, this turned into Blount's disease, which is caused by a local disturbance of growth of the medial aspect of the proximal metaphysis and epiphysis. So, through a lovely combo of genetic and mysteriously environmental factors, my tibias are curved, and my knees bend a bit in the wrong direction.

While it's not a severe condition, it's also not something I could ignore if I wanted to really commit to running. Once I understood how the condition was affecting my performance, I learnt to run differently, in a way that worked for me. On the plus side, because my tibias are curved, my calves look amazing. People often comment on them – and want to touch them – thinking I built them up through running. While this is partly true, the reality is that the physical anomaly I was born with is the biggest contributor to my sexy 'runner's calves'.

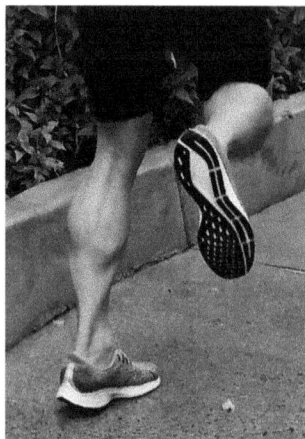

Throughout my life, I've never used my physical impairment as an excuse for underperforming in my sporting activities. In fact, as my 'bent' lower legs were functionally shorter, I held the area boys record for the 'sit and reach flexibility test'. In classical ballet, *genu recurvatum* can be visually appealing and may even be desirable to some people.

My daughter, who is a cross-country runner, says I shouldn't tell people I have leg problems. She thinks it could become an easy excuse to fall back on when I don't perform and reach my goals. Well, I'm going to set the record straight right now: my bilateral legs are no longer a disadvantage. Why? Because I've adapted and learnt to work with what I have. I did this by frequently performing the 'naked' running workouts I described earlier.

Sometimes a Disability Can be a Superpower

I no longer see my bilateral leg impairment as a disability because, in my case, it's not. It simply provides an opportunity for me to do things a little differently. By reframing my condition in a positive light, seeing how my friends and clients comment on my prominent calf muscles, and learning to compensate through specific training strategies, I was able to overcome my inherited impairment.

However, in high school, I didn't know that my bilateral leg issue was causing the shin splints I experienced during every big run, so I just learnt to embrace the suck. If I had to walk, so be it, as long as I finished the race. I would tell myself, *It's okay to walk, but quitting isn't an option. Unless you break an ankle or have a heart attack, you've got no excuse to quit. You keep going, no matter what. Keep moving those legs. Don't stop. Think about the finish. You're running for yourself, but you're also running for the school. Don't let yourself down. Don't let everyone else down. Keep moving!*

I don't know exactly how that mentality got ingrained in me, but I still hold it to this day. One of my own favourite running mantras I've developed continues the 'keep moving' mindset: "I'm not quite the fastest runner of the bunch, but I can run far, and that's my superpower." It's both fascinating and amazing how a supposed deficit can become a pocket source of positive power!

Don't Let Nothin' Hold You Back

As the overweight Fat Doc with congenitally curved lower legs and bend-back knees, I had many reasons not to exercise. For me, the discovery of running was a revelation and a lifesaver.

In our family, others have used the power of running to overcome obstacles. One of my relatives, Geoff, has autism spectrum syndrome (autism) as well as attention deficit hyperactivity disorder (ADHD). The combination of these two developmental disorders has significantly impacted his intellectual, behavioural, psychological, and social development. However, one aspect of his life that autism hasn't affected is his physical endurance. Geoff had the limitation *and* unique talent of being able to maintain one single pace for a long time. During high school, he represented his area in cross-country at two state-level cross-country championships. Running on a variety of courses, terrain, and weather conditions helped Geoff's adaptability and improved his concentration.

However, learning to run can be difficult for people with physical and psychological challenges. Physical impairments can affect running dynamics, and mental health and developmental issues can cause problems with motivation and the ability to adhere to a set running course. These challenges can become sources of psychological stress for both runner and coach.

In Geoff's case, teachers noted improved concentration, greater engagement in learning, and reduction in behavioural problems after he completed a moderate intensity, short-to-medium length (15-minute-plus) run. His parents noticed the same improvements, as well as increased confidence and greater independence in self-care and organisation skills. Running is the gift that keeps on giving!

Why Wouldn't I Prescribe Running?

Given the many benefits of running for both mental and physical wellbeing, why aren't more medical professionals prescribing it as a modality and treatment for chronic illnesses? In my experience, there are several reasons for this.

Firstly, at medical school, there's rarely any formalised training around specific exercise modalities. Modules around exercise generally fall under the sports medicine and rehabilitation medicine specialties.

Secondly, the material taught at medical school is often outdated due to the rapid advances in technology and understanding as well as the delayed publication and subsequent dissemination of scientific running research. Essentially, students and teachers aren't working with the latest information.

Finally, many medical professionals don't feel confident prescribing running to patients due to inherent concerns about direct and indirect injuries. There are actually many exercise screening tests, such as the APSS, which help to mitigate the risks of recommending running to clients who might be susceptible to injury. However, in many instances, doctors simply don't run themselves, so they're less likely to prescribe it to others.

To some people, exercise may seem too low-tech, too non-medical, and too simple to be prescribed by a medical professional. It may not satisfy patient expectations around why they see a doctor. They want a script or an operation – they don't want to be told they simply need to move one foot in front of another.

Running as Both a Lifestyle Practice and Therapy for Medical Professionals and Clinicians

Clinicians are often the cornerstone of medical care in multiple areas, including emergency and inpatient wards, preventative care, and outpatient settings. Thus, there are a myriad of opportunities to incorporate running as a primary and secondary preventative strategy for cardiovascular disease.

Further, to prevent serious health problems, including cardiovascular complications that can lead to death, among highly stressed clinicians, it might also be prudent for medical schools to include aerobic activities as lifestyle and primary preventative measures at a grassroots level.

Who knows? In a parallel universe where these measures were present at med school, it might not have taken me until age 39 to evolve into the Run Doc.

How to Overcome Common Barriers to Running

When I prescribe running as a viable alternative to medications and psychotherapy, I'm often met with excuses or barriers. However, many of these are actually misconceptions that can best be handled by empowering clients with factual knowledge.

Common misconceptions about running include:

1. "I'm too old to run." – Apart from those with cardiovascular instability, almost everyone can run, no matter their age. In fact, there's good evidence that running can help prevent the occurrence of many chronic diseases, thus, increasing 'healthspan' (the absence of disease).

   Human studies have also shown that running improves telomerase inhibitor activity (and prevents telomere shortening), which helps slow the ageing process. In fact, a systematic review of seven studies involving 939 participants found that aerobic exercise (such as running) for more than six months had a significantly positive impact on telomere length.[32] So, running really is the 'elixir of youth'.

   Further, running techniques can be modified by reducing speed or altering the activity. For example, older adults can jog 'naked' on soft terrain, such as grass, to reduce their chances of falling or injury.

2. "I might have a heart attack while running." – While this complication may occur in those with latent cardiovascular disease, such as coronary artery disease or arrhythmias (irregular heartbeat), regular runners actually experience lower prevalence of cardiovascular complications. The occurrence of cardiovascular complications while exercising can be minimised by conducting the pre-exercise APSS questionnaire.

3. "Running will ruin my joints." – The most common barrier cited is the misconception that running contributes to worsened osteoarthritis. With the exception of severe osteoarthritis, running can actually improve musculoskeletal function, and each foot strike can promote the maintenance of cartilage and the integrity of tendons and muscles. As mentioned, when I compared the radiology of my own knees from before running and now, they were slightly improved. For me and many others, running hasn't caused any joint damage whatsoever.

4. "I don't have time to run." – As discussed previously, running as little as 20 minutes daily can actually save us time through improved efficiency and efficacy in our daily lives. Sorry, but the time excuse just doesn't stack up.

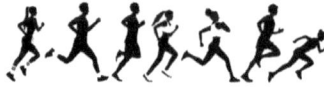

Do You Agree Now That Running is for Everyone?

From Team Hoyt to my relative Geoff to me and my 'crooked' bilateral legs, we've covered several examples that give strength to the idea that running is for everyone. It's a simple modality that's suitable for most ages and physical and intellectual disabilities, with enormous potential to improve wellbeing across the board, saving lives.

Currently, running is an under-utilised modality. It's both a helpful lifestyle habit for busy clinicians, carers, and anyone else and a powerful therapy. If you're not running regularly, there's no better time to start than now.

Run Doc Tips

1

Running is suitable for all ages, genders, orientations, and most body types. You can run at any pace and on any surface.

2

Common perceived barriers to running include age, cardiovascular health, and joint concerns. However, running is for (almost) everyone.

3

Running prescription should be emphasised in medical school.

"When you feel you have been pushed to your limits, ask yourself, 'Why did I start?', and you will be able to push to the end."

– The Run Doc

CHAPTER 7

SURMOUNTING THE INSURMOUNTABLE (OVERCOMING OBSTACLES)

How we perceive an obstacle in our mind's eye matters. You can jump over a molehill with ease, but seeing a mountain in place of that same molehill can significantly affect your ability to complete the task. Conversely, underestimating the gravity of a mission can also affect your ability to complete it.

I entered the 2023 Ultra-Trail 50 kilometre (UTA50) with high expectations. Six months prior, I had achieved a 60-minute PB for the 2023 Six Foot Track Marathon as well as a lifetime road marathon PB at the 2023 London Marathon two weeks before. Approaching the UTA50, I had high hopes and expectations of running a respectable and competitive time. I started the race conservatively, pacing my friend and student, Dr Ken, from the start at Scenic World Katoomba down the Giant Stairway to the bottom of the Three Sisters (9 km). After the first checkpoint at Fairmont Resort (16 km), due to a combination of overconfidence and a strong shot of caffeine from a gel, I redlined (overstretched physiologically) on the next three downhills, passing around 20 competitors.

Sadly, by the 19-km mark, after 900-metre elevations, serious leg cramps set in. Thoughts of dropping out of the race surfaced, and, in my mind, completing the UTA50 became an insurmountable mission. But, as I reflected on my 'running why' and visualised my 'Why Tree' (a visual collective of all my running whys, hanging on a tree like bright, colourful decorations on a Christmas tree) I was able to successfully turn my negative perceptions around and complete my C goal, which was to complete the race two hours before sunset. I was also delighted to see that Dr Ken had completed his race safely in a respectable time for him. Really, the race is only over *if* you decide it is.

Med School Was a Marathon I Almost Didn't Complete

Medical school has a huge dropout rate in the first year for multiple reasons. For starters, the study load is massive; the subject matter can be dense, and stress levels can skyrocket if poorly managed. However, sometimes people quit for more specific reasons.

Without going into too much gruesome detail, the anatomy room is responsible for a lot of people abandoning their medical degrees and never looking back. The pungent stench of formalin isn't something you *ever* forget, and that's just the olfactory, let's say, inconvenience. When you actually have to start pulling body parts out of plastic tubs, it's a whole other sensory experience. If that *is* too much detail, I apologise. Anyway, you can probably imagine why countless students have fainted in the anatomy room and why so many decide that medicine might not be for them after all.

Remember, a medical degree takes six years to complete (or it did when I was studying), which can really test some people. If you study commerce, you can be in and out in three years. Even dentists are done and earning a nice income after five years. Think about it – six years of high-speed lectures, anatomy room nightmares, and stress-inducing exams. It's no wonder many don't see it through to the end. I was able to handle the horrors of the anatomy room better than some, but I failed in other areas.

When I flunked a paediatric clinical exam, I was devastated. I was in my fifth year of uni, and I thought I was starting to get a handle on the whole med school experience, but this failure brought me right back down to Earth. Thankfully, it wasn't the end of the world – yet. I could still take a supplementary exam and redeem myself.

So, I figured out where I went wrong, prepared myself for a second swing at success, and resat the exam. Afterwards, I bought a bottle of Smirnoff and sat at the beach with my now wife, waiting for the moment of truth. Following the results, I would either be drinking that vodka in celebration or commiseration. Obviously, I was hoping for the former. Finally, as the sun was setting, I received a text message – the results were in. "Congratulations…" *Yes!* I had passed. I opened the bottle, feeling good, thankful that I had no sorrows to drown that day.

I knew I wasn't going to be a paediatrician, so I would never have to perform another clinical exam in that field again. Still, the failure rattled me a bit. It showed me that mistakes can be made, conditions can be misdiagnosed, and consequences can be real. As medical professionals, people's lives are in our hands, and we can't leave any room for error. Following my failure, I understood this better than ever. My failure and redemption exemplifies the quality of grit that Rocky Balboa sums up too well in *Rocky Balboa*…

"It ain't about how hard you hit. It's about how hard you can get hit and keep moving forward. How much you can take and keep moving forward. That's how winning is done!"[33]

Ultimately, I learnt a valuable lesson and was able to recover from a major setback. Importantly, I managed to stay in the race.

I've Stacked It More Than a Few Times

While I rarely get injured – touch wood! – injuries are an inevitable part of running, especially when you're really pushing yourself. During one race, I rolled my ankle so badly that I couldn't help but scream in pain. No one was close enough to come to my aid, but I'm sure my yelling carried for miles. As I sat on the ground, nursing my sprained ankle, negative thoughts raced through my head. *I've really done it this time. This is going to put the brakes on my training. I'm not going to be able to run again for… who knows how long?*

After a couple of minutes, I stood up, and, although I was in agony, the pain wasn't unbearable, so I started walking. I told myself that if walking was tolerable, I could increase my pace to a jog. If jogging didn't cause me to collapse in an emotional heap on the trail, I could start running again. Once I realised my running days were far from over, I felt a lot better.

So what if I sprained my ankle? As long as nothing was broken, I could keep going and finish the race, even if it meant walking. Injuries can occur during any event, and you have to be prepared to face them when they do. How will you react when injury strikes? Will you let the negative emotions dominate your thoughts and actions? Or will you find a way to push through the pain and finish the race?

Ten days before the 2023 Six Foot Track Marathon, I sprained my ankle quite badly. I had recently bought some bone conduction sunglasses. If you're unfamiliar with bone conduction technology, I'll quickly explain. 'Bonephones', instead of transmitting sound through the ear canal, use vibrations to send audio through the user's skull. Amazing, right? What will they think of next? So, I was on my morning run, sunglasses on, running through a shady area. Due to the tint on the shades, everything was quite dark. On top of that, the glasses were affecting my depth perception. Did I stop to take the sunglasses off? Nope. Did I at least slow down? Of course not! Eventually, I misstepped, and my ankle reaped the consequences.

Ten days out from a marathon, and I could barely walk. If I went to a doctor, they would likely tell me to stop running until the race. They might even tell me to skip the race altogether. Luckily, I was prepared to do my own diagnosis and prescribe a sensible amount of running in the lead-up to the Six Foot Track. If race day came around and I could only hobble, I still had a chance of finishing the race.

When race day did come around, my ankle wasn't feeling too bad. It wasn't 100 percent, but I could run on it relatively comfortably, which meant I wouldn't have to hobble my way along the track. Bonus!

The first 30 kilometres went well. I was cruising along, and my injury wasn't giving me too much trouble. However, after the 30-km mark, my ankle started to tell me who was boss. But it was only a twinge, so I pushed the complaint aside and kept running. At the 40-km mark, my injury reared its head in a big way. Suddenly, a minor twinge had become crippling pain. Of course, I didn't stop, but I did have to nurse my ankle through to the finish line. It was rough, but I got there. Not only did I finish the race, but I got a 70-minute PB for the course.

Sure, I could have dropped out when my injury flared up, but, physically, I knew I was capable of finishing the race. The real challenge was the mental resistance. The mind-body connection is powerful and when you tell your body who's boss, there are few limits to what you can achieve.

Also, you'll be happy to know that I've stopped wearing sunglasses in shady areas. I'm not eager to make the same mistake twice.

Every Great Success Starts With a Vision

As a doc, I've found visualisation to be a useful tool for not only me but also my patients. For example, if someone in their 50s who's metabolically challenged comes to my office, visualisation can help them make some all-important lifestyle changes. Often, these people have high blood pressure, elevated cholesterol, diabetes, and they love their dessert, their unhealthy snacks, their wine – or all of the above. Generally, they'll say they don't like exercise, don't like to sweat.

So, depending on their situation, I get them to think about their why and visualise certain things. For example, I might say, "Can you visualise your kids growing up? Do you want to see their high school graduation? Do you want to be here to see them graduate university? Do you want to see them get married? Can you imagine yourself holding a baby in your arms as you become a grandparent?" If the answer is yes, their eyes might start to water. "Do you want to experience all of this in the future?" If the answer is yes again, I keep going. "Do you want to be alive and healthy and able to hold that baby?" When they answer yes, we discuss healthy habits and how we can make their vision a reality.

I use the same technique with my running students. In this case, I might get them to visualise winning the prize money, standing on the podium, getting a pat on the back from their friends, eating a celebratory meal – whatever motivates them.

Let's take my friend, colleague, and student, Dr Ken, for instance. His goals are relatively simple: he wants to be healthy, and he wants to finish. However, during the Six Foot Track Marathon, Ken stacked it on the way down to Coxs River and had a nasty rolled ankle injury. For the race, he got a DNF, and the event traumatised him for some time.

In his next race, which was the UTA50, his aim was to finish. I volunteered to pace him, but he declined the offer. So, instead, I said I would be waiting for him with a cold beer at the finish line. To get him through the race, I told him to visualise the beer and the meal we would have together afterwards (and we did enjoy our Asahi together at the end!).

The Power of the Why Tree

Let's talk about the Why Tree. What is it? For starters, it's more than just a term I coined. The Why Tree is a visual, tangible, and mental reminder of our core values around running, as well as our life goals.

Before each race, I construct a Why Tree:

1. **Visual** – I imagine my top three reasons for running, for example, enjoyment of completion, for the bling, for my mental health.

2. **Tangible** – Using the five senses, I form a strong mental picture, for example, a strong hazelnut latte, a beer, driving my favourite sports car, the smell of my partner's perfume.

3. **Memorable** – 'Why' is the homophone of Y, and most trees that we're familiar with have a similar structure, so every time I come across a tree, any tree, it helps generate a strong mental (Why Tree) picture.

By constructing a Why Tree before each race, I run with the mental image of the most important things in my life, each one hanging from the tree. Basically, I'm never in doubt about *why* I'm running. I have clear goals, in running *and* in life, and when I'm tired, struggling, and feel like giving up, I can use my Why Tree as a constant reminder and motivator. It works every time.

The first time I used my Why Tree was in the 2020 Canberra marathon. The last 10 kilometres of any marathon

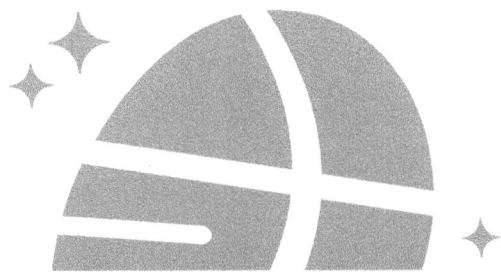

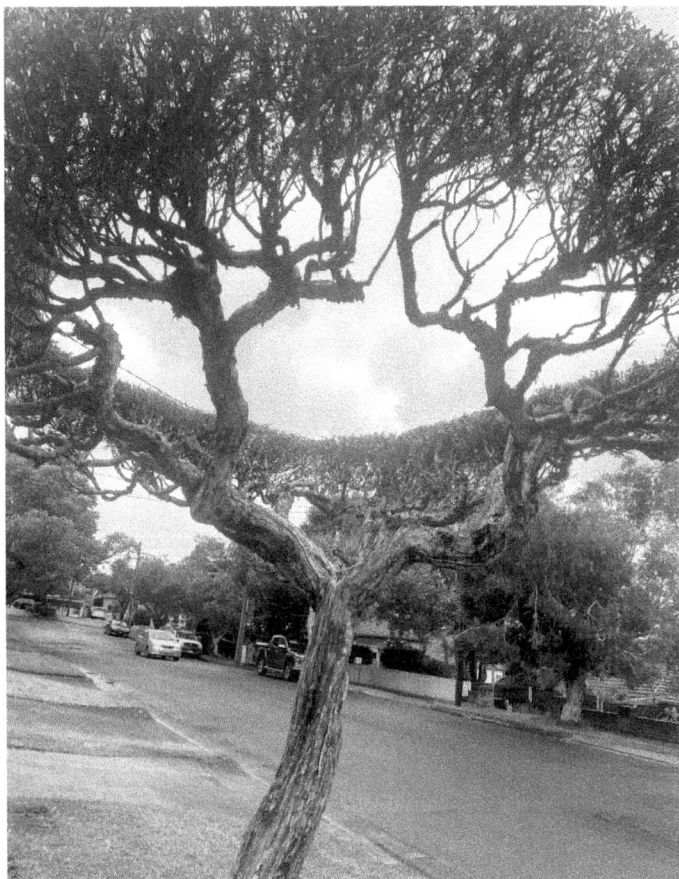

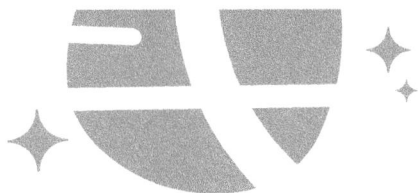

Construct your own
Why Tree.

are always hard, and I was struggling. In front of me, someone was wearing a shirt that said 'RUN DIPG', referencing an organisation that raises money to fight diffuse intrinsic pontine glioma (DIPG). So, I locked in on DIPG, put it on my Why Tree, and kept running with purpose.

Now, you don't want to put too many things on your Why Tree, as it can get a little cluttered. I usually limit myself to four to five items, and most of them are important people in my life. In the Canberra marathon, I had my grandmother, my mother, my daughter, and RUN DIPG all figuratively hanging from my Why Tree, and I kept cycling through these four things. I wasn't even paying attention to my pace; I was just trying to get to the finish line. Whenever the effort got too taxing, I focused on my Why Tree, visualising what will happen, what I want to happen, and what has happened in the past. It's an extremely powerful and motivating tool, and I want to share it with the world.

A Mistake I'll Only Make Once

During my 29th marathon, the people around me were convinced I was dying. It was my first race since the COVID pandemic, so I was excited to be running again. I was carrying some pickle juice in my pocket in case of cramps. I was also carrying some beet juice – this is important.

At the 28th kilometre, I got hit with the cramps, so I pulled out what I thought was my pickle juice and chugged it down. Instantly, I knew I had made a mistake. Whatever I had just consumed didn't taste like pickle juice at all. Clearly, I had drunk the beet juice by accident. *No, no, no, no, no... No, it's good. It's all good.* But it wasn't. The thing is, when you're on the 28th kilometre of a marathon, beet juice isn't what you want to be drinking. In fact, it irritates the stomach and can cause you to – well, you'll see.

Even though a battle was raging in my gut, I persevered. I felt like I was going to chuck. However, I managed to push through to the 37th kilometre before I couldn't hold it in any longer. I stopped and threw up on the track, and, because beet juice is red, it looked like I was vomiting blood. Other runners stopped, looking very distressed, and asked if I was okay. Generally, vomiting blood is a pretty serious symptom, so, naturally, they thought I was dying. I managed to get them to keep running; however, one guy insisted on calling an ambulance. Convincing him that the red liquid pouring from my mouth was just beet juice and not blood took some effort, but he finally left me alone.

On top of everything else, I still had the cramps. My stomach was empty because I had just ejected its contents onto the track, and I didn't bring any food with me. The rest of the race was going to be rough. Even if I'd had food, I don't think I could have stomached it without chucking again.

I was dehydrated and salt-depleted, but I had to finish the race. People who shouldn't have been passing me *were* passing me, and some even offered to run with me. That's how much I was struggling. Several times, the volunteers offered to call me an ambulance, but I politely declined. I was determined to finish the race, even if it meant walking.

The final 5 kilometres were shocking – my slowest ever. In the end, I did finish the race, although I looked like the walking dead by that point. Dad used to say, "Son, it's okay to make mistakes, but don't make the same mistake twice. If you continue to make the same mistakes, you're an idiot." He may have said it more politely than that, but you get my point. Since that fateful day, I've never mistaken beet juice for pickle juice again, and I intend to keep it that way. Lesson well and truly learnt.

Run Doc Tips

1

Running obstacles provide us with opportunities for growth, both physically and mentally.

2

Every success starts with a vision. What's decorating your Why Tree?

3

As my father says, it's fine to make one (running) mistake, but don't repeat it.

"Stay true to
your running course,
and success will follow."

– The Run Doc

CHAPTER 8

FINDING YOUR FLOW

The COVID-19 pandemic significantly impacted my march towards achieving one of my ultimate running goals: qualifying for and running the Boston Marathon.

Up until 2019, I had been making constant progress on my marathon personal best, going from 4 hours 32 minutes to 3 hours 33 minutes, but my training stalled, ultimately, in a good way.

Before COVID, I felt constant pressure to achieve a time goal in every subsequent race instead of enjoying the process. However, during the pandemic, I discovered the joys of virtual races as well as long runs on my treadmill (and running my local trails), which gave me the freedom to dissociate by watching a movie or a running documentary or listening to a running podcast, reducing the rate of perceived effort. It was during one of those long runs that I discovered my running flow.

One Subject Lit a Spark Within Me

At university, we were forced to do a lot of subjects that were very dry, many of which seemed to have no relationship at all to becoming a medical professional. For example, we had to learn the anatomy of a flatworm, study dull biochemistry, and do a lot of pipetting experiments. While these subjects were boring to many of us, they were necessary for people who had come directly from the arts and weren't science-oriented, so I understood why we had to do them.

In among the dry, boring topics, there were unexpected gems. One of the subjects I really enjoyed was ICBS (introduction to clinical behavioural studies). The subject covers human communication, psychological processes, and how the mind works. I developed a strong interest in that area, especially the topic of how the mind can affect the body. In the first lesson, we discussed the biopsychosocial model, and it was a *wow* moment for me. *Wait, our biological, psychological, and social beings are all linked?* For me, the subject provided revelation after revelation.

Studying ICBS more than made up for the dryer subjects I had to endure and opened my eyes to the interconnected nature of every part of us and everything around us. To effectively communicate with someone, we need to understand so much about them, such as their environments and previous experiences. I quickly realised I had an aptitude for ICBS, and I scored my best mark at university in that subject. Although many of my peers had high IQs with superior intellect and analytical abilities, they weren't always adept at communicating with people in the styles and at the levels that best suited each individual. I, however, dove into the behavioural science aspect of medicine wholeheartedly, and it has become a big part of what I do.

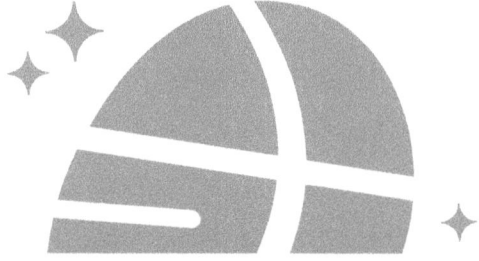

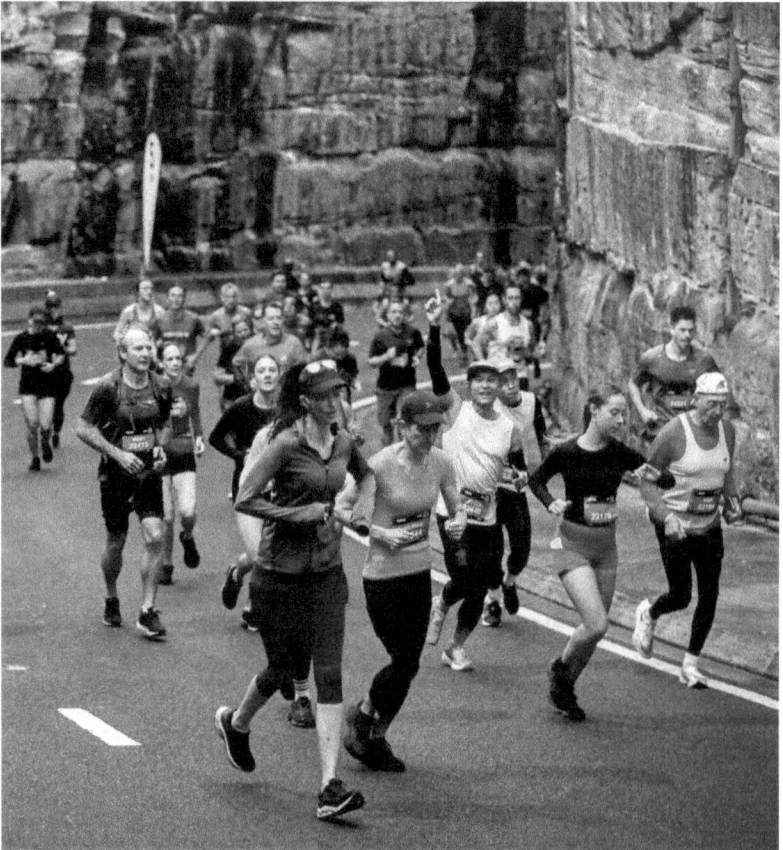

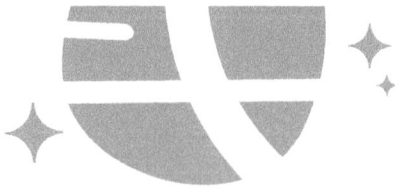

Jenson doing pace duties at the 2023 HOKA 10 km in Sydney.

The Mind, Body, and Heart Connection

The countless ICBS tutorials no doubt sowed the seeds that would later sprout into the premise that running has the power to connect and reinvigorate the mind-body-heart connection. I believe this culminates in the *running flow* state.

Running doesn't just empower the mind with enriching chemicals to create an optimal neuronal state. It doesn't just act as an anti-ageing remedy for the body. Running also has the power to grant control to the central governor, which, in turn, gives us ultimate control over our bodies. It's a classic case of mind over matter.

Everyone Knows Men Don't Have Panic Attacks

I left high school as a top student but when I arrived at med school, I was just another face in a sea of other top students, many of whom were much more accomplished than me. Studying medicine was difficult – of course, it was never meant to be easy – and the whole experience was a bit of a rude shock. Was I in over my head? Had I entered a race I couldn't finish? At the time, I was starting to think so.

On top of that, after spending my high school years surrounded by boys, I was suddenly at a co-ed school. Girls everywhere! A whole new world opened up to me, and I felt like I had to make up for lost time. I wanted to look good, so

I took up running again. I even persuaded Dad to buy me a treadmill, which was expensive back then. However, being the tough dad he was, I knew there would be conditions, and I was right. "If I get you this treadmill," he said, "I want my investment to be worthwhile." He was a business guy, so, naturally, he had to justify his investment. "I want you to promise me you'll run every single day for a year straight – no exceptions."

The challenge was set, and I agreed to Dad's tough conditions. If I failed, I would need to pay back the $2000 he had spent on the treadmill, which wasn't an option. So, I ran when I was sick; I ran when I was tired; I ran when I felt like I couldn't run another step. I ended up running every day for *two* years straight, technically paying him back with interest.

During that time, I was at my lowest weight ever, but I wasn't at my fastest. When it comes to running, fit doesn't always mean fast. The initial healthy lifestyle and running had helped me lose a huge chunk of adipose tissue (fat), but I was yet to build sufficient muscle mass to become a strong runner. At 63 kg, I ran a slower half-marathon than I eventually did at 65.5 kg because the extra 2.5 kg wasn't just extra weight – it was lean muscle.

After my two-year running streak, I continued to run for relaxation, which may seem ironic. But when you're undertaking a highly stressful activity, such as trying to earn a medical degree, intense physical activity is a great way to keep yourself sane. At med school, I felt totally out of my element, but running helped me relax and avoid having the pressure and doubt overwhelm me too much. But I definitely had my moments.

For instance, conducting clinical exams used to give me full-blown panic attacks, which isn't something you want to see in your doctor. You know... the calm, collected, confident professional, who's supposed to be responsible for your health and wellbeing. I knew that panicking in front of my patients wouldn't inspire confidence in my abilities as a budding medical practitioner, so I had to find a solution. While some people resort to drugs to stay calm and relaxed during exam- inations, I didn't see that as a viable, or sensible, option. Yet I had to do something. Every time I started an examination, I felt like I was on an episode of *Thank God You're Here*. If you ever watched the show, you'll know what I mean. In every episode, participants were thrown into an improv situation in front of a live studio audience and had to improvise their way through the scene. That's what clinical exams were like for me. I felt like the audience was watching and judging my every move, which would have been fine if I'd had any confi- dence in what I was saying or doing.

The preclinical work was easy – just memorise the anatomy of an earthworm and whatnot – but walking into a room to meet a patient who's experiencing a medical condition is something else. Within five minutes, I needed to examine the patient, accurately assess the situation, and present the case.

Suddenly, I understood why my GP wanted to hospitalise me for a rash that we ended up curing with cornstarch when I was a kid. Likely, he lacked confidence in his abilities as a doctor and panicked, just as I was panicking in every examination I attempted.

At the time, I didn't know that what I was experiencing were panic attacks. Why? Because Chinese don't have panic attacks – that's why. If we had problems, we dealt with them; we certainly didn't *panic*. I was a man; I had to be strong, and I couldn't show any weakness. *What's the big deal about a bit of high blood pressure? And heart palpitations are usually benign. Nothing to see here, and certainly nothing to worry about, right?* In hindsight, I clearly was experiencing panic attacks, but I didn't label them as such until I reflected on the situation much later.

So, during med school, the night before a clinical exam, I would get anxious and struggle to sleep, which didn't help the situation. An hour or so before an exam began, my heart would start to palpitate, and chest pains followed. When an examination started, the anxiousness would overcome me, which, of course, affected my cognitive skills, adding *more* stress to the situation. On top of that, even though I was a singer – more on that later – I hated the sound of my speaking voice. Yeah, I was dealing with a few confidence issues, but, finally, I found the solution to everything.

Because I wanted to sound more professional, I bought a voice recorder and a book of scripts that outlined what to say during an exam, and I recorded myself talking. I did this often and would play back the recordings, which sounded more professional the more I practised, making adjustments to my diction where necessary. Essentially, I was acting. But after a while, I began to believe the words were actually coming from me. At a certain point, I guess they were. Mum used to tell me to pretend until I didn't have to pretend anymore, and it was great advice – because it worked. With time, practise, and a little make-believe, the examination-fuelled anxiety that had almost crippled me faded into the background. Finally, I could function; I sounded professional, and, importantly, my talking voice didn't bother me anymore.

I hadn't felt anxiety like that in a long time, but the thought of tackling the UTMB 100 – a 100-mile (160-km) ultramarathon through the Alps – scared the shit out of me. As the day of the big race drew closer, more and more butterflies filled my stomach. But they were *good* butterflies. It wasn't crippling anxiety I felt but pure excitement. That's the big difference between me now and me then: I've learnt to embrace the fear and let it fuel me to success. Instead of panic freezing me in place, I now have an unlimited well of positive energy to draw from. I won't ever let fear hold me back again.

I bet you're itching to know how I went in the UTMB 100. Did I complete the race? Was I right to be excited? Or should I have given in to fear? I'm sorry to disappoint, but that's a story for another time.

Do You Want to Achieve Flow? Here's How

When my clients or running students ask me what I do to achieve the flow state, I usually refer them to my tips on running meditation. Occasionally, someone will confide that they had an extraordinary workout, where time and space became dimensionless, an almost out-of-body experience. What they experienced was the 'runner's flow'.

My flow hit rate is around 10 percent. During one in ten runs, the entire workout or a significant portion becomes effortless, pleasurable, and even relaxing compared to other workouts. It's not easy to achieve, but you can get there.

My tips to achieving running flow include:

1. Run at LSD (long slow distance) pace.

2. Alternatively, use the run-walk method.

3. Set a running time, not a running pace.

4. Stick with a regular breathing pattern and use the strategies in the 'How to Practise Mindfulness Meditation the Run Doc Way' section in chapter two.

5. Smile.

6. Finally, my top tip is to treat reaching the flow state like learning to whistle. Don't try to force it. Instead, go with the flow!

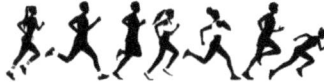

How Doctors Get Their Untidy Handwriting

Have you ever wondered how doctors get their untidy handwriting? Are they just born scribblers? Or is it a style they develop over time? When I got to university, I found the answer.

At the beginning of med school, I walked into a lecture hall filled with people much smarter than me. I was top of my class in high school, but now, among the best and brightest at the University of New South Wales, I was average at best. Admittedly, I felt intimidated and overwhelmed.

The lecture was on the anatomy of the upper limb. Of course, it was the good old days of slide projectors, and we couldn't access the content later online like students can nowadays. Instead, we had to furiously take notes so we didn't miss a thing. The problem was that the professor was talking really fast, almost as if he were sprinting to the end of the lecture. Slide after slide appeared on the screen before quickly flicking away.

Until that moment, my penmanship had been perfect, my handwriting immaculate. But I couldn't write neatly *and* jot down enough information to have a chance of understanding the topic, so I picked up the pace. I once prided myself on my penmanship. However, in that one-hour anatomy class, my handwriting went to shit and never recovered. So, if you've ever wondered where doctors get their untidy handwriting, now you know.

In the age of multi-functioning mobile phones with high-resolution photography, I wouldn't have been so anxious to scribble every word uttered from the lecturer and perhaps may have retained my copperplate handwriting.

Get Your Mental Toolbox in Order

Certain subsets of the running and exercise community love David Goggins. They believe that the 'no pain, no gain' mentality and learning to work with pain are the only ways to success. Personally, I prefer US trail runner, Courtney Dauwalter's, 'pain cave' method.

Dauwaulter, a two-time winner of the UTMB and Western States 100, attributes her success to embracing the pain cave – acknowledging when a rough patch occurs and learning to work with the brain (ego) to process the pain. She uses 'digging the pain cave' to describe training her body and mind to tolerate new levels of discomfort.

I use the same method to unite the mind-body-heart axis to boost my performance in both running and life.

Gaining My Independence and My Future Wife

When I reached my fifth year of uni, I still didn't have a lot of life experience. I was living with my parents, and Mum was taking too good care of me, as Asian mothers do. Eventually, I realised that I had to move out of home, experience life, and learn to look after myself – so I did.

I learnt how to wash clothes and cook again. Although most of my recipes involved a rice cooker, I was still cooking for myself, often on the run. Say what you will about the quality of my meals, but I became a master of fast cooking. During this time, I also started to develop more of a social life, which led to me meeting the woman who would eventually become my wife.

In the 90s, karaoke bars were still a thing. Difficult to believe, right? For us, karaoke was very liberating. We would get up on stage, hold the mic, and sing our lungs out. We didn't even need to sing well, as long as we got up there and gave it a go. Even though I was socialising more, I didn't go out often, nor did my future wife. However, on this fateful night, we both decided to attend a mutual friend's birthday party at a karaoke bar.

When we all sat down at a table, a girl sat next to me. She was well-dressed and smelled really good. Eventually, I got up and sang a song; then she sang a song, and, before we knew it, we were up there singing together. It was a special moment that filled me with positive emotions, so I asked her out. My singing must have impressed her because she said yes, and we've been together ever since.

Even back then, I had the mental toolkit necessary for effectively processing my emotions and staying calm under pressure. That night, I was able to confidently make the first move and score a companion for my most important race – the race of life!

Run Doc Tips

1

One running spark lit a fire in me and gave me
a taste of the mind-body-heart connection.

2

Achieving running flow isn't common
but can be very rewarding.

3

Developing a good mental toolkit through running
can help with many other aspects of life.

"The sprinkling of criticism can add fire to your determination for success."

– The Run Doc

CHAPTER 9

RUN TO PROGRESS, NOT TO IMPRESS

Recently, I attended my younger son's school cross-country carnival. I saw him try his best, run with good form, and finish with a smile on his face. When he got home, he told me he had come first. Clearly, he didn't know I had been spying on him. While he didn't get first place, he did get a ribbon for amazing progress during the year, improving from 48th to 25th place in 12 months. The school presented the ribbon at a weekly assembly, and my son was proud of his achievement, as was I.

The allure of progress, no matter how small or significant, provides us with an internal driver to continue our running. Both the expectation and achievement of progress have fuelled me for much of my running journey.

As the Fat Doc, I found several reasons to continue my running habit:

1. Health-related progress in terms of improvements to my waist circumference, weight, and blood pressure.

2. Subjective improvements to my overall energy levels, vitality, and cognitive speed.

3. Improvements to my sleep habits and overall duration and quality of sleep, likely contributed by running *and* reduced on-call commitments.

4. Objective improvements to stair climbing ability. Gradually, I felt like I was floating up the stairs and was no longer breathless at the top.

5. Subjective compliments from clients and work colleagues about how much happier and younger I looked.

6. Finally, my times for my five laps of the Bert Oldfield Oval consistently improved.

Indeed, I perceived that running was saving my life from premature coronary artery disease and stroke, as well as providing improvements to my ability to be a husband, father, co-worker, fundraiser, medical specialist, and researcher. Ultimately, I ran for progression, not to impress others.

New Home, New Discoveries

One of my grandmothers was the good cop, and the other was the bad cop. I'm sure you can guess who my favourite was. One grandmother would scold me if I did something wrong, while the other would scold *her* for scolding me. It was an interesting dynamic; that's for sure. Between me and my brother, who's three years younger than me, I think I

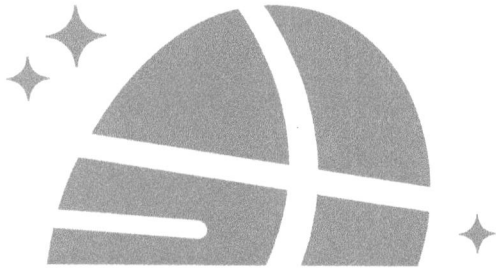

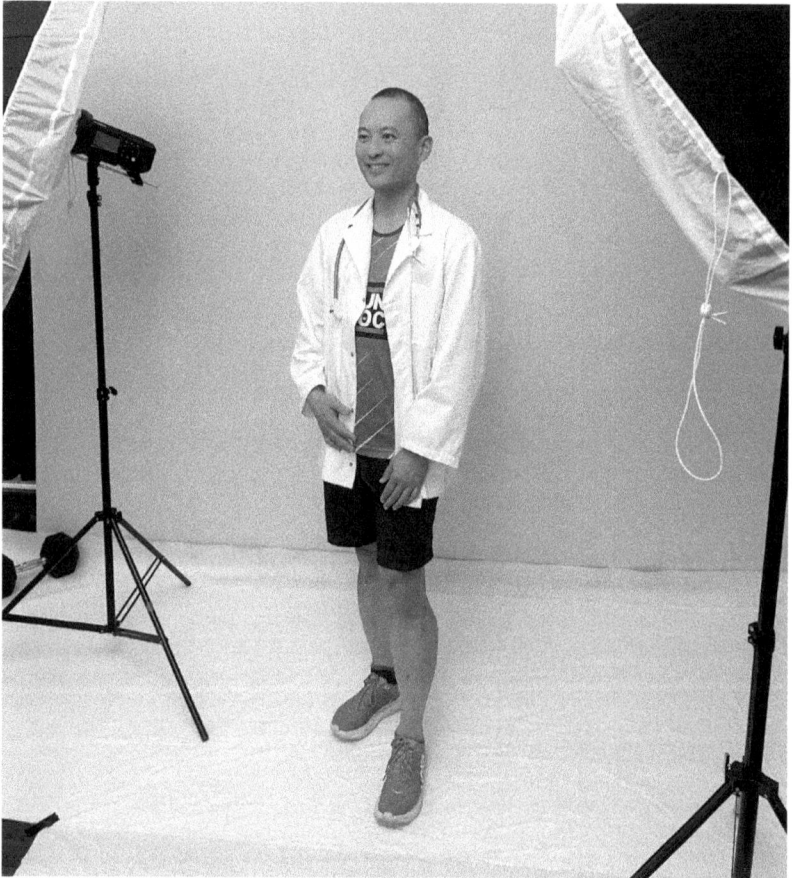

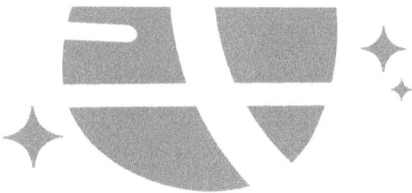

The Run Doc thrilled with his latest photo shoot.

got the better deal. He was raised by our working parents – no offense to working parents. I *am* a working parent, so I understand the struggle. But my grandmothers were very attentive, whereas my parents weren't, which must have made my brother's formative years difficult. Like I said, I think I got the better deal, but, hey, I could be wrong.

Growing up in Hong Kong, I had a traditional Chinese upbringing, so sports weren't really encouraged, which was unfortunate for many reasons. At age 6, I left my grandmothers' care and went to live with my parents and brother. Finally, when I was 7, we moved to Australia, which had a much more sports-oriented culture. Perfect. During the move, I didn't understand what was happening, but I knew something wasn't right. For instance, why were my grandmothers crying at the airport as they saw us off? I knew then that we weren't just going on a holiday. We were going away for a long, long time.

My parents were opportunists, and they saw an opportunity in emigrating to Australia. They also took the opportunity to drill the classic immigrant story into our heads, the one they believed they were living. "We gave up so many things to bring you to Australia, so you better work hard." I did work hard, but I also liked playing video games, so Mum was constantly questioning what I was doing. Why wasn't I studying? Why wasn't I doing my second hour of piano? *Why* was I playing video games? My mother, she was a tigress – the boss of the household.

My father was a busy man, but he gave me his time when he could. He recognised early that I had some ADHD-like tendencies, and he did his best to nurture those traits. Video games were one outlet. I also enjoyed watching TV, particularly a show called *It's a Knockout*. The program had contestants compete in a series of insane challenges. During the competition, they were tested; their weaknesses were poked, and they were thrown into the fire. Sometimes, they would literally jump through fire. To win, contestants didn't have to be the fastest or the strongest; they simply had to be smart about how they approached each challenge. If someone rushed, they would usually make an error and end up stacking it. If they were too slow, the faster contestants would beat them. It was all about balance. *It's a Knockout* taught me that winning isn't just about strength or speed. It's also about strategy.

Why I Run – to Progress, Not Impress

The moment I discovered the motto, "Run to progress, not to impress, run to progression, not perfection," I knew it captured the essence of what running is all about.

From day one of my running journey, I've documented and reflected on each run with apps such as Runkeeper and, more recently, with my Strava journal. At the end of each run, I always give myself a mental high five, no matter how

I went, and a mini compliment, focusing on what I did well. I also critically evaluate each running workout and look for areas to improve. Comparing current results to past efforts provides ongoing accountability to make meaningful improvements. If you're part of a running group, you can even compare yourself with others for additional accountability and motivation.

Three years ago, I started journalling my thoughts about running as well as discussing other life hacks on my Facebook blog, which, as of writing, has over 72,000 followers. I also began sharing my journey on my Instagram, which now has over 12,000 followers. These RUN DOCSTERS (Run Doc followers) help keep me accountable in my training and my races. Also, having a mass of interested people following my progress is great when motivation starts to wane or when I enter the pain cave. In challenging times, I can draw on their presence for fuel to keep pushing forward.

Run to Progress, Not to Perfect

Many people have asked me why I place a greater emphasis on progressive mini goals rather than massive achievements. The answer is simple: humans are much more receptive to praise over ridicule and success over failure. So, for example, rather than aiming to shave, say, 60 seconds off a 5-km PB, it might be more realistic and achievable to aim for a 10-second improvement. Baby steps eventually lead to big outcomes, and constantly hitting targets, no matter how small, keeps the inner fire of motivation burning.

As I mentioned previously, when I race, I always set several goals of differing magnitudes, for example, an A, B, and C goal. Of course, I would love to hit my A goal every time, but it's not always possible. We're running to progress, not to perfect, remember? While we can strive for amazing results, we won't always hit those targets, so we must be content with progression in whatever form it takes.

Sprinting My Way to Defeat

In primary school, we had weekly swimming lessons, which introduced me to the idea of regular exercise. We didn't do any advanced training, just the basics. Basically, we learnt enough to avoid drowning.

However, once I moved to Riverview College, a Catholic school for boys, sport became a much bigger part of my life. At Riverview, they valued sport as much as – if not more than – academics, which was confusing for someone who'd had a traditional Asian upbringing. But I quickly embraced the cultural contrast. Sport was something I could get excited about.

I quickly realised that knowing how to not drown in a pool wasn't enough. If I didn't want to lose face, I had to learn how to swim well. So, in the middle of year 6, Mum enrolled me in the Carlile Swimming school, which was a humbling experience. Because my skills were, let's say, less than advanced, I had to start in the bottom class. I was literally in the pool with babies. But once I proved myself to be a more capable swimmer than an infant, I moved up to the next class. Progress! Finally, after three months of persevering, improving my skills, and moving up the levels, I was able to join the Carlile swim squad, which was a huge achievement.

Squad training was tough. Sessions were 90 minutes long, nonstop, and super intense. The coach pushed us hard, and I pushed myself harder, ending most sessions spewing in the shower. Clearly, I wasn't holding back.

In year 8, I qualified for the school swim team, which was a big step up from learning the basics in the baby pool. However, my parents were getting busier and busier, and they didn't have time to keep up with my training commitments, so I never got the chance to represent the school in competition. There's definitely an unfulfilled dream there, but it's fine. I soon discovered other sports.

I needed something to do during the winter, but my parents didn't want me to get my head smashed in playing rugby, so I settled on cross-country. During training, our coach would make us do two laps of the school. That may not sound like much, but Riverview was *massive*. It was practically its own suburb. So, when the coach assigned us two laps, we weren't running a short distance; we were doing about 2 kilometres every time.

During cross-country, I always pushed myself, and I was fast, but I kept making the same mistake. Whenever we started running, I would sprint to the front of the pack, going all-out. By the end of the run, I was gassed, survival jogging to the finish line, with everyone charging right past me. I usually finished in the bottom two.

When Mum arrived to pick me up, she only ever saw the end of the run, which, admittedly, looked bad for me. "Jenson, what's wrong? Why are you struggling so much? I don't think you should do this anymore. You look like you're about to die." If she had seen me sprinting earlier, she would have understood. Instead, she missed my mad dash at the start and assumed something was physically wrong with me. Ultimately, I had neglected to strategise, which was something I knew was important in sport. So, I continued to try to sprint my way to victory.

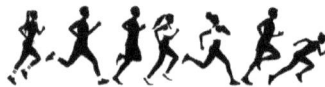

A Manifestation of My 2023 UTMB Race Experience

My cross-country captain daughter taught me a valuable tool for my UTMB preparation: manifestation. What do I mean? I'm talking about visualising the successful completion of the race prior to the event. Let me explain.

On my treadmill runs, I often watch Jeff Pelletier's YouTube video of his 2022 UTMB race experience with his wife, Audrey. Doing this helps me imagine myself in the same position, on the same course, running the same race. I visualise myself tackling the most difficult parts of the UTMB. I imagine myself entering my pain cave and running with light feet, good technique, and a relaxed body and mind.

In June 2023, I took my visualisation a step further by travelling to the UTMB course and experiencing Chamonix (the start and finish), Les Contamines, Les Bains, Les Houches, as well as Courmayeur (the race's halfway point). By becoming familiar with different parts of the course, I lessened the chance of any surprises on race day.

As I write this, I'm sitting on a balcony in a Les Houches chalet on a warm summer's evening. Throughout the day, periodic showers and storms accompanied my exploration of the UTMB course, and wandering clouds now partially obscure my view of Mont Blanc. Here, 1200 metres above sea level, I sit and ponder life and my running why, feeling great appreciation for all the love I've received from family, friends, and RUN DOCSTERS (my blog supporters). I'm thankful for their kindness and support on this journey. As I close my eyes and breath in the crisp alpine air, while birds chirp in the distance, I manifest a happy UTMB journey, built upon a foundation of running to progress, not to impress. Through visualisation, I experience the joy I'll receive as I smile during the most difficult points of the journey, knowing that my supporters and my late mother, who shares a birthday with the UTMB, will be smiling with me.

Run Doc Tips

Running for progression and not perfection
helps you better focus on your short-term goals
and align them with your long-term goals.

Run to impress yourself, not anyone
else. The sense of intrinsic motivation
to succeed is more powerful and
sustaining than anything extrinsic.

As my daughter often reminds me, "You have
to manifest it before you can achieve it." I
would also like to add the importance of grit.

"Never regret a run.
Good runs give happiness,
bad runs give experience,
worst runs give lessons,
and best runs give
memories."

– Anonymous

CHAPTER 10

THE JOURNEY FROM SUBHEALTH TO HAPPINESS

As the Fat Doc, I was living in a subhealth state, neither healthy nor diseased. Frankly, I was probably an inch from developing a heart attack (like Dr A) or a stroke, but I managed to grip the steering wheel of life, turn it around 180 degrees, and head back up the healthy highway. Being 20 kilograms overweight (literally carrying two bags of 10 kg rice on my body!) and in a chronically stressed state, I wasn't functioning at my full human potential as a father, brother, clinician, or researcher.

However, the discovery of running, both as a therapeutic measure for my metabolic syndrome as well as a lifestyle measure helped me lose 20 kg of fat and then regain 4 kg of muscle. I commenced my journey as a healthier human being and springboarded into a part-time career as a masters athlete. With an improved physical and psychological state, I became happy again and regained my 'mojo', filling with happy hormones each time I ran.

Getting Fit Wasn't a Sprint – It Was a Marathon

When you're a busy professional, you need to set targets and hold yourself accountable. So, when I started running again, I set myself the goal of completing the Sydney Morning Herald Half Marathon, an annual road race that takes runners to many of Sydney's iconic landmarks, including Hyde Park. I

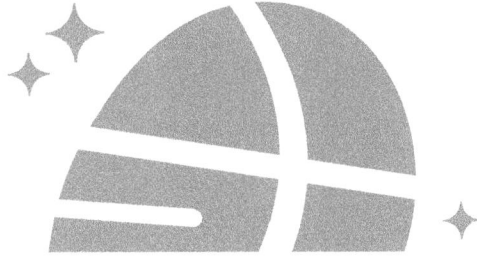

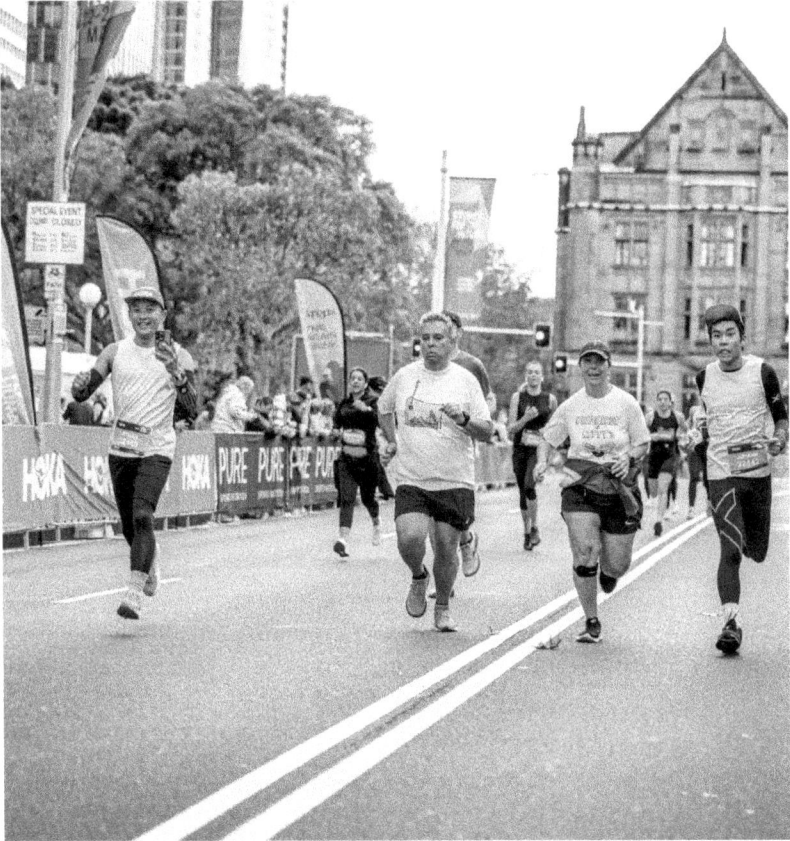

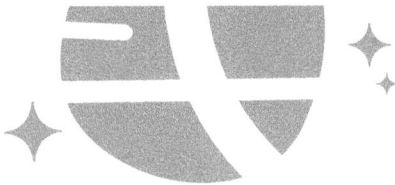

Happy finishing line snap from the 2023 HOKA 10 km event in Sydney, Australia.

had set a clear objective (complete the race), but how would I stay accountable? I solved the accountability problem by setting another target around money raised. I fundraised *hard*, and, on race day, I was named as one of the top five individual fundraisers. Donors had pledged a lot of money to see me finish the race, so, for me, failure wasn't an option.

When fundraising for the race, I had to include a statement about why I was raising money and entering the event. In my statement, I said: "I want to be happy, healthy, and raise awareness of general health, men's health, and mental health." I put it out there, and the message resonated with people.

I also wanted to tell people how I felt, what I was experiencing, and, hopefully, inspire them to take up similar health and fitness challenges. So, I turned to the internet and started blogging. That's when I introduced myself to the world as the Run Doc. When I started my blog, I didn't want to write wordy essays or create dry, clinical, lifeless content that may be educational but not necessarily fun or inspiring to read. Instead, I simply jotted down my thoughts, hoping to inspire at least one person. If I did inspire just one person, I would have been happy. Then I thought, *What if I could inspire ten people?* That would be great. *Wait, what if I could inspire 100 people? What about 1000 people?* My eyes lit up at the thought.

When I thought about what I was creating as the Run Doc, I started to draw parallels between it and singing. As a singer, I couldn't just stand up on stage and sing the lyrics. There was more to it than that. I also had to tell a story and send emotion to the audience. Without emotion, a song is little more than some music with a bunch of words attached. However, when you pour emotion into a song – or a blog – it affects people on a deeper level. If you're really good, you can move and inspire them.

Once I started my blog, something unexpected happened. Initially, I thought blogging would be a one-way communication, but I was wrong. As I shared more of my thoughts and my journey – the struggles, the triumphs, and the raw truths – people started writing to *me* with words of encouragement.

As a professional, I'm expected to hide myself from the world. I'm not supposed to express myself in a way that reveals my personality or my humanity. In the professional world, sharing too much of yourself is frowned upon. It dispels any illusions, lowers you in the eyes of others, and leaves you vulnerable to attack. But none of this is actually true. When you're open and honest about your experiences, people begin to feel like they know you, and you can earn their trust much more easily. If I want to help and inspire people, they need to know my journey. They need to know all of it, from couch potato to ultramarathon runner and, let's be honest, proud, self-confessed running addict. Without knowing someone's journey, how can we truly understand and appreciate where they are now?

My blog served as an outlet to express myself in a way I couldn't in my day-to-day work as a medical professional. Singing didn't become my career, but at least now I have other outlets for my inner thoughts, emotions, and personality, including this book.

Am I worried about oversharing? No way! I'm sharing my unfiltered fitness journey because I know that others are still in their Fat Doc stage, and I want to show them what's possible. If I do receive criticism for oversharing, I'll simply run it off, and the negativity will drip away like the sweat from my brow.

Don't Run Happy, Run Happier

As well as generating a high level of accountability around my own running, my Run Doc blog brings joy and happiness, inspiring others to achieve greatness and reach their personal best.

I recently coined the phrase, "Don't run happy, run happier!" to support one of my pillars of running for healthy ageing. 'Run happy' comes from the motto of the Port Macquarie Running Festival, home of the Treble Buster (half-marathon, 10 km, and 5 km all completed in one morning), which I've completed four times. Why do I prefer 'run happier'?

Australian running champion, Robert 'Deek' de Castella, reminds us to find a higher purpose for our running – which is exactly what I've done. From running to achieve and maintain a healthy state of mind and body, I've now transitioned to challenging my mental and physical state. Also, by disseminating the Run Doc primary health promotional message that running can be a key prevention strategy for cardiovascular disease, I also hope to save lives.

So, why not run happier?

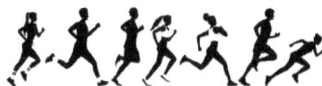

My First Running Coach Wasn't Who I Expected

In my life, four women have made a massive impact: my grandmother on my dad's side, my mother, my wife, and my daughter.

My daughter is like a mini me in feminine form, which is difficult for me to accept sometimes. Like me, she's determined, prefers to save face, works hard, especially when facing an adversity, and doesn't like to admit defeat. She also shoots straight from the hip, telling it like it is. When I was in, shall we say, less than impressive shape during the COVID

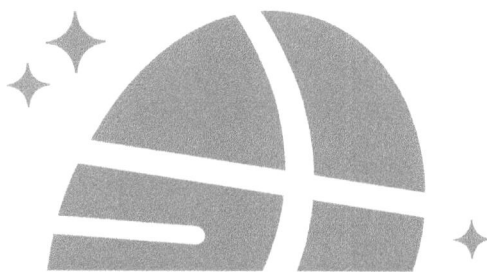

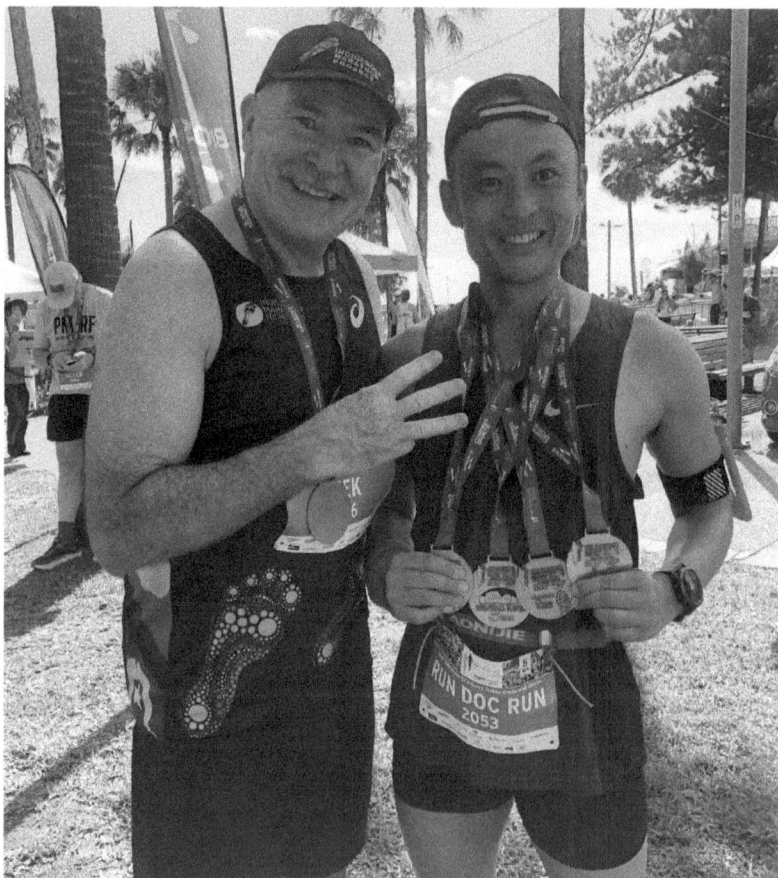

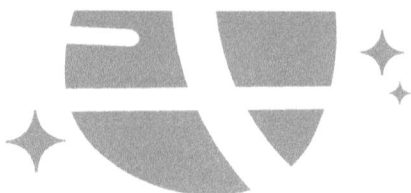

The Run Doc meeting up with Robert 'Deek' de Castella upon completion of the Port Macquarie Treble Buster.

pandemic, she told me, "Dad, you're fat." Just like that. No honey, no sugar, just the unsweetened truth.

I didn't know how to respond. "Oh, okay, thanks. What do you mean?"

"Your belly has gotten bulgy since COVID."

"Okay, cool."

With her, I know I'm always going to get the hard truth. She doesn't hold anything back.

Technically, she was my first real running coach. When I was obese and out of shape, we were running around the oval at the dog park, where I was meant to be training *her* for a 2-kilometre cross-country run. I lasted about 300 metres before I had to double back and pretend that stopping to time her was really important. From that moment on, I knew I wasn't coaching her; *she* was coaching me.

She ended up qualifying for the 2017 IPSHA Cross Country Carnival, representing her school (Abbotsleigh), coming 14th out of about 200 runners, and advancing to the area level CIS Carnival. In the lead-up to the race, it had rained heavily, so the course was muddy. Have you heard the saying, "The hills are your friend?" Well, on this day, the muddy fields were her friend. In those harsh conditions, she managed to outsprint some of the faster girls, finishing the race covered in mud, and she did it all with very little training. It had to be genetics, right? In my mind, the genetics came from me, but my wife says they came from her because she also represented her school in cross-country. She's wrong, however. The genetics definitely came from me.

My daughter was representing her all-girls primary school, where she was usually expected to be clean and neatly dressed, with her hair in a ponytail, so seeing her cross the finish line covered in mud sparked a remark from her principal. "The dirtier she is," she said, "the harder she tried." She was right. My daughter had qualified for the next race because she was prepared to try much harder than many of the other girls. Unlike some, she didn't have any formal training. But we did *informally* train, and, on race day, she executed the plan perfectly.

As a makeshift coach, I felt strong pride in what she had achieved. I had managed to teach her a few things, but, in the end, she taught me much more than I taught her.

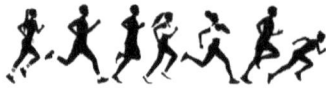

My Biggest Supporter – a Shoutout to Ken

Dr Ken is a bariatric surgeon, friend, colleague, running student, and one of my biggest supporters on my own running journey. Every day, he deals with overweight and obese people, and he would be the first to tell you that running is the best form of exercise for many of his patients. Unfortunately, many of those patients aren't motivated to exercise or adjust their diets, so, instead, they turn to surgery for a solution. Like I said, he has been – and still is – one of my biggest supporters and motivators.

When I could barely run 100 metres without getting puffed out, he said, "Why not try 1 K?"

What is he thinking?

When I could run 1 kilometre, he said, "Why not try 5 K?"

This man's insane.

When I achieved 5 kilometres, he said, "What about 10 K?"

Come on now…

"What about a half marathon?"

Is he serious?

"What about a *marathon?*"

All right, maybe he's onto something.

Back then, running a marathon seemed totally crazy, but Ken was right to encourage me because every time he pushed me, I succeeded and grew as a runner and as a person.

Whenever I achieved a goal, he would throw down the next challenge. "What about UTMB?"

"Ken… I can't do UTMB. People die in that race."

"Yeah, but you'll make it."

"Are you sure?"

"I'm sure."

"All right!"

Before I knew it, I had qualified for the UTMB and was preparing to head to France to hopefully not die running one of the most daunting ultramarathons in the world.

With all that said, when it comes to his own running, Ken is fairly conservative. He's not taking any big risks. But when it comes to *my* running, suddenly, he's got an all-in attitude – which is exactly what I need to motivate me. And when Ken pushes me to hit that next level, it helps his own running too. It's practically a form of visualisation for him. He can't imagine himself, say, running an ultra but if he pushes me to do it and I succeed, the goal seems more achievable to him, and he's able to take himself to that next level too. It's an unorthodox strategy, but I can't argue with the results.

Run Doc Tips

1

Goals worthy of praise take time
and steady practise.

2

Don't just run happy, run happier!

3

Sometimes, your best running lessons
come from the most unlikely sources.

"My running philosophy:
1. Pick a goal that
   intimidates you.
2. Work steadily towards
   that goal.
3. Watch yourself become
   a better version of your
   current self."

– The Run Doc

CHAPTER 11

DREAM FURTHER THAN YOUR LEGS CAN TAKE YOU

When I signed up for the 2022 Ultra-Trail Australia 100-km trail ultramarathon – or the UTA100 – I had no idea how long that distance would feel physically or, more importantly, psychologically. Before the UTA100, the longest trail ultramarathon I had completed was the 2022 Six Foot Track Marathon – a tough race with several river crossings. But The UTA100 was over twice the distance and elevation!

During the 100-km journey, I had to pull out many of my mental tricks, including letting go of any mental constraints and visualising myself crossing the finish line. I also had to overcome the control of my 'central governor' to achieve my running freedom and complete the distance.

When I achieved my goal, my dream of completing a 171-km (with 10,000 m elevation) UTMB came to life, and my next epic goal was set. So, during every workout, race, challenge, and before I closed my eyes at night, I fervently manifested a vision of me crossing the finish line after a gruelling run through the mountains, with tens of thousands of spectators cheering me on!

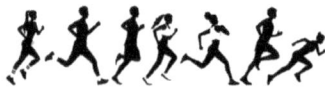

Great School, But There Was One Big Problem

When we moved to Australia, I went to a small Catholic school in North Sydney: St Mary's Catholic Primary School. The principal and teachers shared my grandmothers' ethos. They were tough but attentive, and I appreciated the structure the school provided. Because my parents were tough but generally *inattentive*, I also appreciated the attention I received.

So, I was attending a great school, but there was one fairly significant problem: I didn't know a word of English. In Hong Kong, I was always among the top students in the class but in Australia, I was right at the bottom. To learn English, we used the Endeavour program, which was a series of fifteen books that got progressively more difficult with each one. While most of my peers were already on book eight, I had to start right from the beginning, so I had some catching up to do. But I was determined. I set myself the goal of finishing that series before the end of the year, which was already half over. But that didn't matter to me. The challenge was set.

As I'm sure you can imagine, making friends was difficult when I didn't know what the hell anyone was saying. I did, however, have a few friends who spoke Cantonese, so I wasn't completely alone. We were all curious to hear what the English-speaking students were saying. Because of that curiosity and FOMO (fear of missing out), I pushed myself to try to learn the language. It wasn't easy, especially in the beginning. While I didn't cry outwardly, I was crying on the inside. Hey, learning a new language is tough. But even though I was struggling, I didn't let myself become a victim of my circumstances. Instead, I read and read and read some more – sometimes five books per night. Luckily, I'm very adaptable, and it wasn't long before the language started to sink in. While I didn't achieve my goal of finishing the Endeavour series before the end of the year, I did get to book 14 and was once again among the top students in the class.

A Tale of Two Doctors

When I finished high school, my parents wanted me to work in the family business with my brother, but doing so would have been at odds with my personality. While they offered to pay me well, I would have to work in an office, performing unfulfilling tasks I wasn't the least bit interested in. I would have felt trapped, *caged,* and I couldn't live like that.

Once I said I didn't want to work in the family business, Dad decided I should become a dentist. Dentists made lots of money, drove nice cars, and, importantly, didn't have to be great conversationalists. Most people don't talk much when they have a hand in their mouth. At that time, I was, let's say, working on my communication skills, so Dad saw the lack of conversation as a plus. We all have our weaknesses, and that was mine. For a long time, I had wanted to be a scientist

– think the Chinese Albert Einstein – so, in that regard, dentistry was appealing.

However, six weeks before I sat my final high school exams, I got really sick. I had high temperatures and broke out in a terrible rash. So, I went to a GP who was a family friend. He was an ultra-conservative doctor, very cautious. After he examined me, he told Dad I needed to be hospitalised. *What?!* Because the doctor couldn't figure out what my illness was, he wanted to play it safe and let the hospital deal with it. Dad wasn't convinced, so he took me to see another GP, Dr Cho. He was ABC (Australian-born Chinese), very cool, and had a different assessment than the first doctor. Dr Cho told us to chill out because my condition wasn't serious. *What?!* We had gone from one extreme to the other. So, what was his remedy? Cornstarch bath and Panadol. That's it. He pre-scribed a cornstarch bath for the rash and Panadol for the temperature. If I didn't improve or got worse, *then* it would be time to go to the hospital. But, for now, he thought I seemed quite well. Guess what? After following Dr Cho's advice, I felt better within a day.

The first doctor was so fearful of making the wrong decision that he took the easy way out and tried to palm me off to the hospital. However, Dr Cho was operating on a whole other level. I was so impressed with his clinical skills that I began to consider medicine as a career. When I thought about how the first doctor had struggled to make a diagnosis or take any responsibility for my treatment, I thought, *I can do better than that.* I had convinced myself that medicine was the right career, but I still had to convince Dad.

"Dad," I said – I was very timid at this point – "can I change from dentistry to medicine?" I explained why I had made this decision, and he responded with a look of complete disapproval.

Finally, after much contemplation, his expression shifted. "Okay," he said, "if you get good enough marks to get into medicine, you can put it as your first selection. *But* I want you to put dentistry second." With a sigh of relief, I agreed. The hard part, convincing Dad, was over; now all I had to do was get really good marks so I could actually get into medicine. Easy, right? I instantly sprang into action, studying hard so I didn't have to become a dentist like Dad wanted. While I knew I would do well, I didn't know *how* well I would do. As it turned out, I got one of the top marks in my school and was the only year 12 from that graduating class to go directly into med school. Most of my peers became lawyers, so I have a lot of lawyer friends. I had made it!

After such a significant achievement, I had a slightly overinflated opinion of myself. Can you honestly blame me? However, when I got to med school, I quickly learnt that I wasn't as special as I thought.

What I Really Wanted to Be When I Grew Up

It may surprise you to learn that I'm a closet extrovert. Or perhaps I'm not so closeted anymore, but there was a time when I was still discovering the authentic version of myself, the one that wasn't repressed by cultural or parental expectations. For instance, I didn't always want to be a doctor when I was young. I almost went down a very different path.

When I was choosing subjects for uni, Mum asked me what I wanted to be when I grew up. I vividly remember my answer: "I want to be a singer." Silence.

Finally, the shock wore off, and Mum spoke. "Son, your father and I sacrificed a lot to bring you here. We gave up our high-income jobs in Hong Kong to come to Australia. We left our home country to give you the best opportunities possible. You're a smart boy, and singers, you know, they don't earn a lot of money. You could do much better."

"But I want to perform," I said. "Singing is my calling." At that time, I truly believed it.

"Why do you want to be a singer?" Mum asked.

"Because I want to have a positive impact on the world. I want to make people happy and inspire them, and singing is how I do it."

Eventually, we came to an agreement. I was allowed to pursue singing as a hobby. Mum even helped get me on stage, usually at charity events. We would get a table, and friends would purchase tickets; then Mum would talk to the event organiser and arrange for me to be one of the guest singers.

Although I'd only had three singing lessons, I was a pianist, and, at age 15, I was teaching younger kids how to play piano. That was another of many moments in my life when I had to pretend until I actually knew what I was doing. I wasn't a trained piano teacher, but I knew how piano teachers acted, so I played the part until I *became* the part. Singing was very much the same. I wasn't a trained singer, but I could certainly play the part, and I did.

My first big performance was at the Sydney Town Hall, which isn't a small venue. I was 22 years old at the time. When I performed, the floor was completely full, and the upper tiers were at about 95 percent capacity. I was pretty much singing to a full house. I sang two songs: 'The National Anthem' and 'Music of the Night', which is my favourite song from *The Phantom of the Opera*. The gig went great, and I was even in several local newspapers the next day.

I also had another amazing singing experience while on a cruise when I was 42 years old. For fun, I entered an on-board competition called 'The Voice of the Ocean'. I didn't expect to do well, so I didn't bother putting any effort into presentation, showing up in T-shirt, shorts, and thongs. Hey, don't judge me. I was on a cruise, after all.

After all 100 of us contestants had sung our songs (I sang 'What a Wonderful World'), the audience voted.

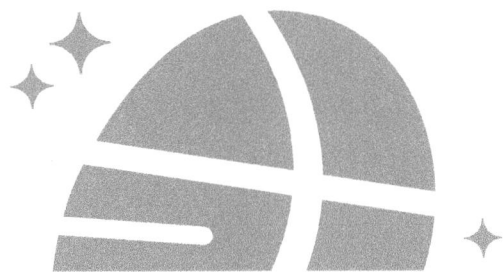

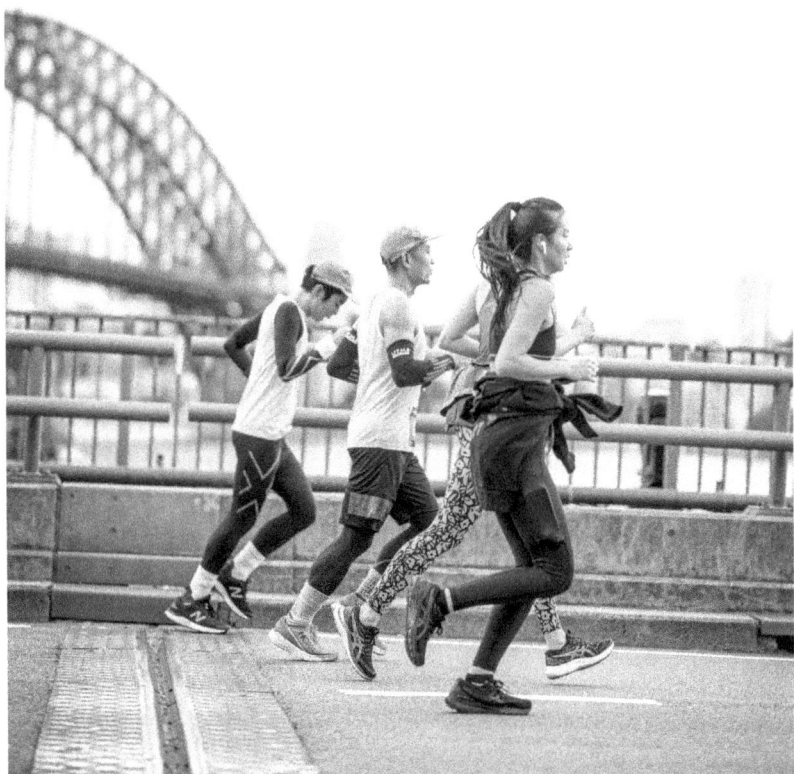

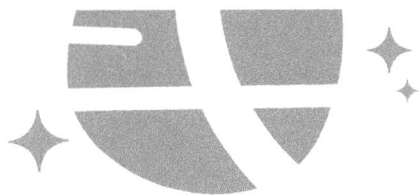

The Run Doc doing pace duties at the 2023 HOKA 10 km in Sydney.

Unfortunately, my family had gone to bed, so I missed out on their votes. I didn't expect much to come of my performance, so I was more than a little surprised when I was announced as one of the finalists. I had made it into the final six. How did this happen? Well, it was an Alaskan cruise, and, honestly, I think I earned a few extra votes for my Australian accent. I sang from the heart, and my performance resonated with that cruise ship audience. What does any of this have to do with running? I was just getting to that.

Firstly, I was so underdressed for the performance because I had been running laps on the upper deck. As I discovered, running provides a nice aerobic base for singing projection. The more I ran, the more I improved my cardio fitness and lung capacity, and the more effortless singing became. When I'm fit and healthy, I feel like my diaphragm is supercharged with unlimited energy, and I can stand up on stage and belt out any song with ease. On the contrary, when we lose our fitness, we often experience a negative flow-on effect into other aspects of our lives. Exercise is about so much more than being physically fit. It's the key to enjoying and excelling at everything we do in life.

My Mentors Made Me Who I Am Today

Throughout my life, I've turned to others for guidance on many occasions. Whether I need advice about my education, career, or running, I've always sought out people who are smarter or more experienced than me to help guide me in the right direction.

For example, when I failed a paediatric clinical examination at university, I found the smartest student in my year group and bought him coffee. We had a chat; I explained that I had stuffed up the exam, and I asked for his advice. He told me I was studying the wrong way, and he explained the *right* way to study. While everyone has their own way of doing things, this guy was as smart as they came, so I took his advice seriously. With his help, I passed the supplementary exam and pushed on with my degree. If I had been too proud to ask for help, I might have failed and been forced to drop out of med school. Thankfully, I knew what I needed to do to have the best chance of success.

When I started my medical internship, I didn't have any good mentors. There were no doctors in the family, so I didn't have anyone I could turn to for advice and guidance. That was part of the reason why the first few months of my internship were so brutal, almost unbearable. I made a lot of mistakes, but we were taught not to ask for help, so messing up was the only way I was able to learn.

Looking back, completing my internship was tougher than running an ultramarathon. I was doing shift work, experiencing night shift for the first time, certifying deaths, putting lines into people, breaking bad news to patients and their families, ringing the boss to say their patient had passed away – it was tough. I had to be sharp at all times, even when blunted by a severe lack of sleep. People's lives were in my hands, and a single mistake could have been catastrophic. The pressure was immense and a lot for a fresh intern to deal with. Still, I never considered quitting. To me, giving up just wasn't an option.

If I'd had a real mentor during that time, I'm positive the whole experience would have been much more tolerable, valuable, and educational. It's not that I didn't want to ask for help; it's more that I didn't know *who* to ask. Sometimes, finding the right mentors is the most difficult part of seeking help. Often, however, the right mentors *are* there if you know where to look.

When I was considering getting my PhD, I reached out to Michelle Peate, a family friend, who had completed her PhD in psychology. I asked her if I could buy her coffee, and she misunderstood the offer at first. "No, no, I'm married," I said. "I just want to pick your brain."

So, we met for coffee, and I explained that I wanted to get my PhD. I asked for her advice regarding whether the goal was achievable. She said I could do it. After all, she had done it, so it was definitely possible. She stressed the importance of hard work and gave me a good understanding of the effort needed to succeed. Once I knew what to expect and had the backing of someone who had already achieved what I wanted,

I was ready to meet the challenge. In 2015, I completed my PhD, and it wouldn't have happened if I hadn't reached out for advice.

When it came to running, and surviving, the UTMB, I couldn't go in blind. I needed a mentor, someone who had successfully completed the race before, to give me the all-important guidance that only comes from experience. So, I reached out to a guy named Wong Ho Chung, who placed sixth in the UTMB in 2019 and tenth in 2021. He was very generous, not only giving me tips but also his training plan. His most important piece of advice was to do more elevation work. I had been doing too much mileage, whereas training elevation was the key to completing the UTMB. Once again, the simple act of asking for help was a game changer for me.

When it came to this book, Dr Catherine Yang, author of *Step on Fear*, was one of the people who spurred me to write it. She was my kids' dentist and whenever I was in her office, she would tell me I had to write a book about running. Being an author herself, she knew what she was talking about. When I was finally ready to write this book, I reached out to Catherine for advice. She has been there, done that, and she filled me in on exactly what to expect. If it weren't for Catherine, her guidance, and her belief in me, I might never have had the confidence to write this book. But here we are!

If you're considering taking on a massive challenge, whether it's completing a PhD, running an ultramarathon, writing a book, or tackling some other monumental feat, reaching out to people who have done it all before will make the experience much smoother, and you'll be more likely to succeed. The guidance of great mentors is an invaluable asset in all aspects of life and should never be overlooked.

Work Hard, Play Harder

The term 'grit' comes from 'grit salt', which is ground rock salt that's used to de-ice roads. When the rock salt is spread the evening before a big freeze, it prevents ice and snow from sticking to the road. Clearly, without grit, in harsh weather, you're going to have problems.

From a psychology perspective, in runners, grit is the learnt quality that prevents them from pulling out of races, even when the going gets tough. It promotes an attitude of persistence and fortitude in the face of adversity.

As I run towards new and exciting goals, I always make sure I accurately and frankly address each workout in my Strava log and share each success on the Run Doc blog. We should all celebrate the attainment of each goal, big or small, because positive reinforcement propels us onward towards our next big success.

Run Doc Tips

1

Setting a massive goal for yourself can be a double-edged sword. However, if you approach it in smaller steps, the task feels much more achievable.

2

Running is a good outlet for both latent extroverts and absolute introverts, as it offers an expression of your running self.

3

Be open to seek the advice of mentors who have climbed those mountains before you.

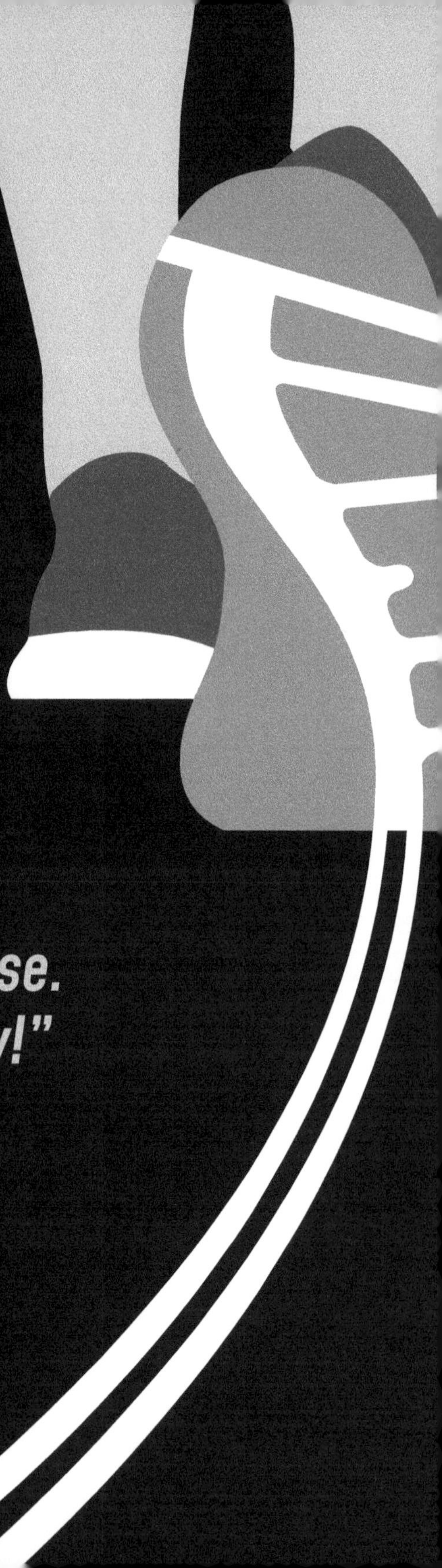

"Plan with purpose.
Act with alacrity!"

– The Run Doc

CONCLUSION

MY MAIN
MESSAGE
TO YOU

At the end of the day, the main message I want to share with you, the reader, is: *there are no shortcuts in life.* I'll admit, I've made mistakes while trying to cut corners in the past, but I quickly learnt that you've got to put in the hard work every time if you want to be successful, in life, running, singing – anything.

If you're unwilling to put in the work, don't expect to be able to consistently perform. Whatever you're trying to be successful at, you must approach it in the right way. Don't look for ways to cut corners. What may appear to be a shortcut will ultimately end up taking you the long way around, towards potential danger.

If you're following the correct process, the results will follow. You don't even need to be thinking about the results. If, instead, you focus on the process itself and doing things the right way, you'll inevitably end up where you want to be.

When it comes to running, I always follow the workouts I design for myself, and I try not to overtrain. Honestly, I don't have time to overtrain, which helps, but I'm always conscious about pushing myself too hard and doing more harm than good. Remember, there are no shortcuts in life. Any goals worth achieving require hard work, dedication, and commitment to the task.

I'll sign off with a quote from my cross-country captain daughter in her thankyou speech to the school…

"I love cross-country because I believe it is not only a wonderful sporting event, but also teaches us about how to approach life. You run into bumps and curves, and can even fall over. But as long as you keep your goal in mind, you will cross the finish line with your head held high."

– My daughter, aged 12

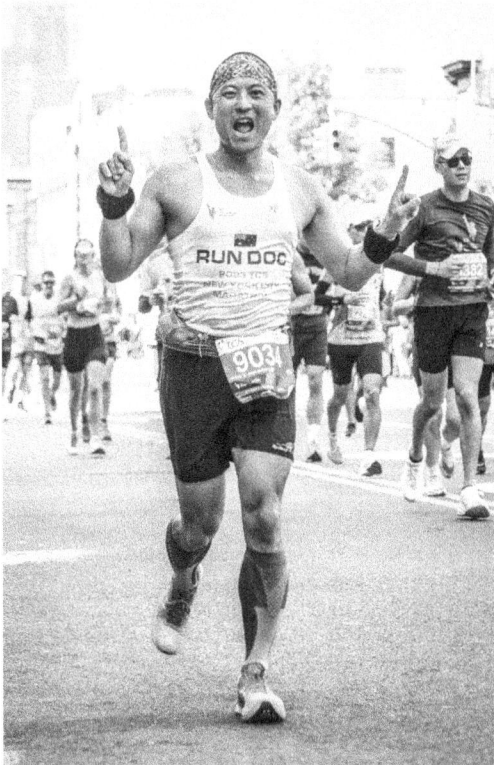

Jenson celebrates the completion of his 40th marathon at New York City (NYC) Marathon on 5 November 2023.

Bonus Content

Dear Reader (RUN DOCSTER),

If you have reached this point of *Trailblazing*, I commend you and give you a mental high five. Well done!

As a reward for your persistence, I would like to share with you my thoughts before the 2023 New York City Marathon.

"My training for this race has been predicated by a fruitful experience at UTMB 2023, a relatively short training block involving progressive 1-km repeats ('Dales Demons'), and recovering from a plantar plate tear."

 Scan the QR code or go to www.therundoc.com.au/bonus to follow my journey and access additional bonus content, including my running playlist.

ACKNOWLEDGEMENTS

I wish to acknowledge my father, who has provided me with many hours of coffee chats about life, the universe, and how to become the 'top 2 percent' of society. When I asked him why not strive to be the top 1 percent, he said, "You should always act like you are number two, chasing the number one position, even if you think you're in front."

Huge thanks to Susan Dean for her inspirational support, Monique, Chloe, editor-in-chief Natalie Deane, Matt, Dani, and Jaz from the Dean Publishing team, who provided an opportunity for me to tell the Run Doc story.

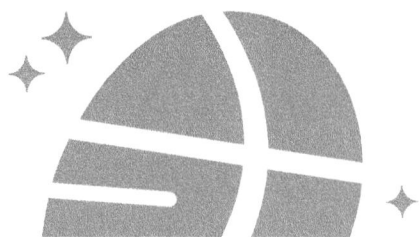

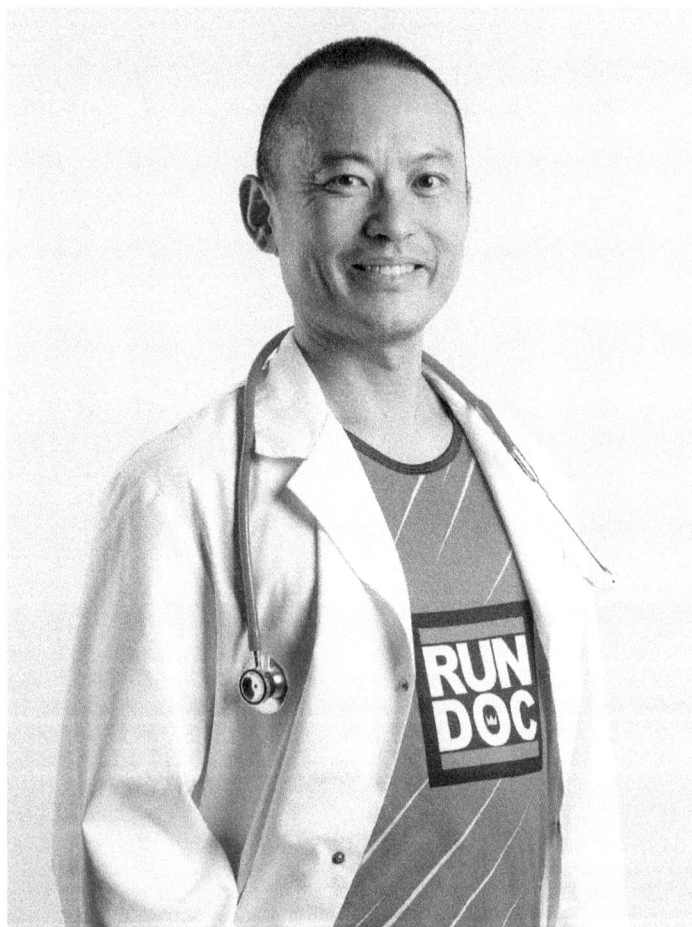

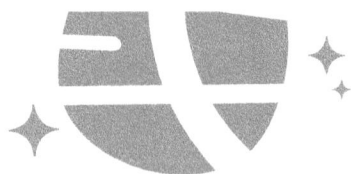

ABOUT THE AUTHOR

Jenson 'The Run Doc' Mak is a healthy ageing and longevity specialist who discovered the elixir of youth through running, transforming himself from the Fat Doc to the Run Doc.

On the precipice of 'subhealth', with high blood pressure, insomnia, work stress, and mental health disorders, he developed a strong desire to better experience the life events of his three children, which drove him to improve his physical and mental health.

As well as being an accomplished runner, Jenson is a clinical researcher, senior lecturer in clinical medicine, and justice of the peace. He's also a certified primal health coach and one of the first to become level three performance development coach in road, trail, and ultra running with Athletics Australia. For leisure, he enjoys singing and reading about psychology.

A Special Request from the Run Doc...

I would appreciate it immensely if you could leave a review of *Trailblazing* on my website.

Website: therundoc.com.au

Facebook: facebook.com/rundoc2run

Instagram: instagram.com/the_run_doc/

ENDNOTES

1   Robbins, T 2022, *If You Can Recognize PATTERNS*, video, TikTok, viewed 8 August 2023, https://www.tiktok.com/@tonyrobbins/video/7149210608959819051?lang=en.

2   Armstrong, A et al. 2022, 'Effect of Aerobic Exercise on Waist Circumference in Adults with Overweight or Obesity: A Systematic Review and Meta-Analysis', *Obesity Reviews*, vol 23, no 8, viewed 2 August 2023, https://doi.org/10.1111/obr.13446.

3   Szortyka, MF, Cristiano, VB & Belmonte-de-Abreu, P 2023, 'Aerobic and Postural Strength Exercise Benefits in People with Schizophrenia', *International Journal of Environmental Research and Public Health*, vol 20, no 4, viewed 2 August 2023, https://doi.org/10.3390/ijerph20043421.

4   Ferguson, JM 2001, 'SSRI Antidepressant Medications: Adverse Effects and Tolerability,' *Primary Care Companion to the Journal of Clinical Psychiatry*, vol 3, no 1, pp 22-27, viewed 3 August 2023, https://doi.org/10.4088/pcc.v03n0105.

5   Liu, PZ & Nusslock, R 2018, 'Exercise-Mediated Neurogenesis in the Hippocampus via BDNF', *Frontiers in Neuroscience*, vol 12, no 52, viewed 14 September 2023, https://doi.org/10.3389/fnins.2018.00052.

6   Erickson, KI et al. 2011. 'Exercise Training Increases Size of Hippocampus and Improves Memory', *Proceedings of the National Academy of Sciences of the United States of America*, vol 108, no 7, pp 3017-3022, viewed 14 September 2023, https://doi.org/10.1073/pnas.1015950108.

7   Piya, MK 2021, 'Improvement in Eating Disorder Risk and Psychological Health in People with Class 3 Obesity: Effects of a Multidisciplinary Weight Management Program', *Nutrients*, vol 13, no 5, viewed 2 August 2023, doi.org/10.3390/nu13051425.

8   Schleppenbach, LN 2017, 'Speed- and Circuit-Based High-Intensity Interval Training on Recovery Oxygen Consumption', *International Journal of Exercise Science*, vol 10, no 7, pp 942-953, viewed 3 August 2023, https://www.ncbi.nlm.nih.gov/pmc/articles/PMC5685083/.

9   Viana, RB et al. 2019, 'Is Interval Training the Magic Bullet for Fat Loss? A Systematic Review and Meta-Analysis Comparing Moderate-Intensity Continuous Training with High-Intensity Interval Training (HIIT)', *British Journal of Sports Medicine*, vol 53, no 10, pp 655-664, viewed 3 August 2023, https://doi.org/10.1136/bjsports-2018-099928.

10 Klein, D, Guenther, C & Ross, S 2016, 'Do as I Say, Not as I Do: Lifestyles and Counseling Practices of Physician Faculty at the University of Alberta', *Canadian Family Physician*, vol 62, pp e393-399, viewed 3 August 2023, https://www.cfp.ca/content/cfp/62/7/e393.full.pdf.

11 Singh, B et al. 2023, 'Effectiveness of Physical Activity Interventions for Improving Depression, Anxiety and Distress: An Overview of Systematic Reviews', *British Journal of Sports Medicine*, viewed 3 August 2023, 10.1136/bjsports-2022-106195.

12   Affes, S et al. 2021, 'Effects of Running Exercises on Reaction Time and Working Memory in Individuals with Intellectual Disability', *Journal of Intellectual Disability Research*, vol 65, no 1, pp 99-112, viewed 3 August 2023, https://doi.org/10.1111/jir.12798.

13   Wang, S et al. 2021, 'Exercise Dosage in Reducing the Risk of Dementia Development: Mode, Duration, and Intensity-A Narrative Review', *International Journal of Environmental Research and Public Health*, vol 18, no 24, viewed 3 August 2023, https://doi.org/10.3390/ijerph182413331.

14   Maffetone, P 2015, 'The MAF 180 Formula: Heart-Rate Monitoring for Real Aerobic Training', *Maff Fitness*, viewed 14 September 2023, https://philmaffetone.com/180-formula/

15   Lee et al. 2011, 'Long-Term Effects of Changes in Cardiorespiratory Fitness and Body Mass Index on All-Cause and Cardiovascular Disease Mortality in Men: the Aerobics Center Longitudinal Study', *Circulation*, vol 124, no 23, pp 2483-90, viewed 18 September 2023, 10.1161/CIRCULATIONAHA.111.038422.

16   Lee et al. 2014, 'Leisure-Time Running Reduces All-Cause and Cardiovascular Mortality Risk', *Journal of the American College of Cardiology*, vol 64, no 5, pp 472-481, viewed 18 September 2023, doi.org/10.1016/j.jacc.2014.04.058.

17   Lautenschlager, NT et al. 2008, 'Effect of Physical Activity on Cognitive Function in Older Adults at Risk for Alzheimer Disease: A Randomized Trial', *JAMA*, vol 300, no 9, pp 1027-1037, viewed 18 September 2023, doi:10.1001/jama.300.9.1027.

18   Jaret, P 2011, 'Exercise for Healthy Skin', *WebMD*, viewed 18 September 2023, https://www.webmd.com/skin-problems-and-treatments/acne/features/exercise.

19   Sherrington, C et al. 2020, 'Evidence on Physical Activity and Falls Prevention for People Aged 65+ Years: Systematic Review to Inform the WHO Guidelines on Physical Activity and Sedentary Behaviour', *International Journal of Behavioral Nutrition and Physical Activity*, vol 17, no 144, viewed 18 September 2023, https://doi.org/10.1186/s12966-020-01041-3.

20   Alentorn-Geli, E et al. 2017, 'The Association of Recreational and Competitive Running with Hip and Knee Osteoarthritis: A Systematic Review and Meta-Analysis', *The Journal of Orthopaedic and Sports Physical Therapy*, vol 47, no 6, pp 373-390, viewed 3 August 2023, https://doi.org/10.2519/jospt.2017.7137.

21   Ponzio, DY et al. 2018, 'Low Prevalence of Hip and Knee Arthritis in Active Marathon Runners', *The Journal of Bone and Joint Surgery*, vol 100, no 2, pp 131-137, viewed 18 September 2023, https://doi.org/10.2106/JBJS.16.01071.

22   Coburn, SL et al. 2022, 'Is Running Good or Bad for Your Knees? A Systematic Review and Meta-Analysis of Cartilage Morphology and Composition Changes in the Tibiofemoral and Patellofemoral Joints', *Osteoarthritis and Cartilage*, vol 31, no 2, pp 144-157, viewed 3 August 2023, https://doi.org/10.1016/j.joca.2022.09.013.

23   Timmins, KA et al. 2017, 'Running and Knee Osteoarthritis: A Systematic Review and Meta-Analysis', *The American Journal of Sports Medicine*, vol 45, no 6, pp 1447-1457, viewed 3 August 2023, https://doi.org/10.1177/0363546516657531.

24   ESSA n.d. *Pre-Exercise Screening Systems*, webpage, viewed 18 September 2023, https://www.essa.org.au/Public/Public/ABOUT_ESSA/Pre-Exercise_Screening_Systems.aspx.

25   Lambrias, A et al. 2023, 'A Systematic Review Comparing Cardiovascular Disease Among Informal Carers and Non-Carers', *International Journal of Cardiology*, vol 16, https://doi.org/10.1016/j.ijcrp.2023.200174.

26   Longman, J 2016, '85-Year-Old Marathoner Is So Fast That Even Scientists Marvel', *The New York Times*, viewed 4 August 2023, https://www.nytimes.com/2016/12/28/sports/ed-whitlock-marathon-running.html.

27   Hollander, K et al. 2019, 'Adaptation of Running Biomechanics to Repeated Barefoot Running: A Randomized Controlled Study', *The American Journal of Sports Medicine*, vol 47, no 8, pp 1975-1983, viewed 18 September 2023, https://doi.org/10.1177/0363546519849920.

28   Noakes, T 2007, 'The Central Governor Model of Exercise Regulation Applied to the Marathon', *Sports Medicine*, vol 37, no 4-5, pp 374-7, viewed 24 September 2023, doi:10.2165/00007256-200737040-00026.

29   Oxford Union 2018, *Eliud Kipchoge & David Bedford | Full Address and Q&A | Oxford Union*, video, YouTube, viewed 4 August 2023, https://youtu.be/Tc00mDtzIJU.

30   Team Hoyt 2023, *Team Hoyt*, webpage, viewed 4 August 2023, https://teamhoyt.com/.

31   White, ES 2014, *File:Team Hoyt in Wellesley.JPG*, image, Wikimedia Commons, viewed 20 September 2023, https://commons.wikimedia.org/wiki/File:Team_Hoyt_in_Welleslley.JPG.

32   Song, S, Lee, E & Kim, H 2022, 'Does Exercise Affect Telomere Length? A Systematic Review and Meta-Analysis of Randomized Controlled Trials', *Medicina*, vol 58, no 2, viewed 19 September 2023, https://doi.org/10.3390/medicina58020242.

33   Stallone, S 2006, *Rocky Balboa*, Metro-Goldwyn-Mayer, California.

www.ingramcontent.com/pod-product-compliance
Lightning Source LLC
Chambersburg PA
CBHW052113030426
42335CB00025B/2960